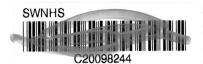
The National Collaborating Centre

for Chronic Conditions

Funded to produce guidelines for the NHS by NICE

PARKINSON'S DISEASE

National clinical guideline for diagnosis
and management in primary and secondary care

Published by

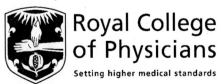

Royal College
of Physicians
Setting higher medical standards

Acknowledgements

The National Collaborating Centre for Chronic Conditions would like to thank Rob Grant, Susan Varney, Ian Lockhart, Lina Bakhshi, Alison Richards, Jane Ingham, Ester Klaeijsen, Nick Latimer and Bernard Higgins for their work and advice on this project.

The Royal College of Physicians

The Royal College of Physicians plays a leading role in the delivery of high quality patient care by setting standards of medical practice and promoting clinical excellence. We provide physicians in the United Kingdom and overseas with education, training and support throughout their careers. As an independent body representing over 20,000 Fellows and Members worldwide, we advise and work with government, the public, patients and other professions to improve health and healthcare.

The National Collaborating Centre for Chronic Conditions

The National Collaborating Centre for Chronic Conditions (NCC-CC) is a collaborative, multi-professional centre undertaking commissions to develop clinical guidelines for the NHS in England and Wales. The NCC-CC was established in 2001. It is an independent body, housed within the Clinical Standards Department at the Royal College of Physicians of London. The NCC-CC is funded by the National Institute for Health and Clinical Excellence (NICE) to undertake commissions for national clinical guidelines on an annual rolling programme.

Citation for this document

National Collaborating Centre for Chronic Conditions. *Parkinson's disease: national clinical guideline for diagnosis and management in primary and secondary care.* London: Royal College of Physicians, 2006.

Copyright

ISBN 1 86016 283 5

ROYAL COLLEGE OF PHYSICIANS
11 St Andrews Place, London NW1 4LE
www.rcplondon.ac.uk

Registered Charity No 210508

Typeset by Dan-Set Graphics, Telford, Shropshire
Printed in Great Britain by the Lavenham Press Ltd, Sudbury, Suffolk

Contents

APPENDICES

REFERENCES

Guideline Development Group members

Name	Job title	Employing organisation	Representing
Carl Clarke	Clinical Advisor	City Hospital and University of Birmingham	NCC-CC
Tara Sullivan	Research Fellow and Project Manager	NCC-CC	NCC-CC
Alastair Mason	Chairman	NCC-CC	NCC-CC
Bernadette Ford	Information Scientist	NCC-CC	NCC-CC
Debbie Nicholl	Health Economist	NCC-CC	NCC-CC
Jill Parnham	Senior Research Fellow	NCC-CC	NCC-CC
Nicole Wilson	Project Manager	NCC-CC	NCC-CC (6 months)
David Anderson (GDG member)	Consultant Psychiatrist	Mossley Hill Hospital, Liverpool	Royal College of Psychiatrists
Angela Birleson (GDG member)	Advanced Practitioner in Occupational Therapy	Occupational Therapy, Clinical Support Services, South Tees Hospitals NHS Trust	College of Occupational Therapists
David Burn (GDG member)	Consultant Neurologist	Newcastle General Hospital, Newcastle upon Tyne	Royal College of Physicians of London
Michael Godfrey (GDG member)	Patient Representative	–	Parkinson's Disease Society
Jacqui Handley (GDG member)	Parkinson's Disease Nurse Specialist	Dorset County Hospital, Dorchester	Parkinson's Disease Nurse Specialist Association
John Hindle (GDG member)	Consultant Physician, Care of the Elderly	North West Wales NHS Trust, Bangor	British Geriatrics Society
Brian Hurwitz (GDG member)	General Practitioner	King's College London	Royal College of General Practitioners
Andrew Lees (GDG member)	Professor of Neurology	Reta Lila Weston Institute of Neurological Studies, Institute of Neurology, University College London	Association of British Neurologists
Doug MacMahon (GDG member)	Consultant Physician (with special responsibility for the elderly)	Royal Cornwall Hospitals NHS Trust	British Geriatrics Society

continued

Name	Job title	Employing organisation	Representing
Robert Meadowcroft (GDG member)	Director of Policy, Campaigns and Information	Parkinson's Disease Society	Parkinson's Disease Society (Attended ten meetings)
David McNiven (GDG member)	Policy and Campaigns Manager	Parkinson's Disease Society	Parkinson's Disease Society (Attended two meetings)
Bhanu Ramaswamy (GDG member)	Consultant Physiotherapist	Walton Hospital, Chesterfield	Chartered Society of Physiotherapy
Julia Johnson (Expert advisor)	Speech and Language Therapist	King's College Hospital London	Royal College of Speech and Language Therapists
TRK Varma (Expert advisor)	Consultant Neurosurgeon	Walton Centre for Neurology & Neurosurgery, Liverpool	Society of British Neurological Surgeons
Ana Aragon (Deputy for Angela Birleson)	Occupational Therapist	Bath and North East Somerset PCT	College of Occupational Therapists (Attended one meeting)
Ira Leroi (Deputy for David Anderson)	Consultant in Old Age Psychiatry	Manchester Mental Health and Social Care Trust	Royal College of Psychiatrists (Attended one meeting)
Karen Durrant (Deputy for Bhanu Ramaswamy)	Superintendent Physiotherapist	Walton Hospital, Chesterfield	Chartered Society of Physiotherapy (Attended one meeting)
David Stewart (Deputy for Doug MacMahon)	Consultant Physician (medicine for the elderly)	Mansionhouse Unit, Victoria Infirmary Glasgow	British Geriatrics Society (Attended one meeting)

Preface

It is almost 200 years since James Parkinson described the major symptoms of the disease that came to bear his name. Slowly but surely our understanding of the disease has improved and effective treatment has been developed, but Parkinson's disease remains a huge challenge to those who suffer from it and to those involved in its management. In addition to the difficulties common to other disabling neurological conditions, the management of Parkinson's disease must take into account the fact that the mainstay of pharmacological treatment, levodopa, can eventually produce dyskinesia and motor fluctuation. Furthermore, there are a number of agents besides levodopa that can help parkinsonian symptoms, and there is the enticing but unconfirmed prospect that other treatments might protect against worsening neurological disability. Thus, a considerable degree of judgement is required in tailoring individual therapy and in timing treatment initiation.

It is hoped that this guideline on Parkinson's disease will be of considerable help to those involved at all levels in these difficult management decisions. The guideline has been produced using standard NICE methodology and is therefore based on a thorough search for best evidence. Because of the unique problems of Parkinson's disease, converting this evidence into recommendations for treatment might have been problematic, but we have been fortunate in having a very experienced and able Guideline Development Group who have interpreted the scientific papers in the light of their considerable clinical experience. I am grateful to them for their hard work and for their expertise.

The guideline includes many recommendations on the use of different classes of pharmaceutical agent, but the recommendations singled out as being of key importance also stress other aspects of management. This is not a negative emphasis based on the problems associated with anti-parkinsonian drugs, but reflects the major role of non-pharmacological aspects of care in this disabling chronic condition. Diagnosis is particularly highlighted. This can be difficult, and while swift assessment by someone with appropriate expertise is important when suspicion of Parkinson's disease first arises, so too is it vital to reconsider the diagnosis if atypical features develop later. The speed with which we have recommended that patients should be seen may seem aspirational, but reflects the importance the Development Group feel should be attached to this. Other key recommendations urge healthcare professionals to be aware throughout the course of the disease of the potential benefits of referral for specialist treatment such as physiotherapy, occupational or speech and language therapy. I would also commend to the reader the excellent section on communication, another area of particular difficulty in this disease.

One of the incidental benefits of producing an evidence-based guideline is that the process highlights those areas in which the evidence is particularly lacking. There are always more of these than we would wish. Towards the end of this document the Development Group has indicated those areas which they believe are particularly deserving of, and amenable to, further research efforts.

Two centuries since its first description, Parkinson's disease remains a huge challenge. We hope that this guideline will not only aid current treatment of the disease, but will also stimulate efforts to improve future management more quickly than has been possible to date.

Dr B Higgins MD FRCP
Director, National Collaborating Centre for Chronic Conditions

DEVELOPMENT
OF THE GUIDELINE

1 | Introduction

1.1 Background

Parkinson's disease (PD) is named after the London general practitioner (GP), James Parkinson, who vividly described many of the clinical features of the condition in his *Essay on the shaking palsy* (1817).[5]

In this work, Parkinson refers to the condition by its earlier name of *paralysis agitans*, a term that captures a peculiar characteristic of the disease, namely the combination of *movement loss* (ie hypokinesia) with *movement gain* (ie tremor at rest) which characterises the condition.[6]

Shaking palsy was named 'maladie de Parkinson' in 1888 by the French neurologist Jean-Martin Charcot. Charcot admired Parkinson's clinical acumen and powers of description, but criticised him for omitting mention of rigidity, which Charcot believed to be a typical feature of the condition.[7]

1.2 Modern definition

PD is a progressive neurodegenerative condition resulting from the death of the dopamine containing cells of the substantia nigra. There is no consistently reliable test that can distinguish PD from other conditions that have similar clinical presentations. The diagnosis is primarily a clinical one based on the history and examination.

People with PD classically present with the symptoms and signs associated with parkinsonism, namely hypokinesia (ie poverty of movement), bradykinesia (ie slowness of movement), rigidity and rest tremor.

Parkinsonism can also be caused by drugs and less common conditions such as: multiple cerebral infarction, and degenerative conditions such as progressive supranuclear palsy (PSP) and multiple system atrophy (MSA).

Although PD is predominantly a movement disorder, other impairments frequently develop, including psychiatric problems such as depression and dementia. Autonomic disturbances and pain may later ensue, and the condition progresses to cause significant disability and handicap with impaired quality of life for the affected person. Family and carers may also be affected indirectly.

1.3 Health and resource implications

PD is a common, progressive neurological condition, estimated to affect 100–180 per 100,000 of the population (6–11 people per 6,000 of the general population in the UK)* and has an annual incidence of 4–20 per 100,000.[8] There is a rising prevalence with age and a higher prevalence and incidence of PD in males.[9]

---

*The size of the average general practice list in the UK.

PD can lead to extensive disability, which affects both the individual with the disease as well as indirectly family and carers. The economic impact of the disease includes:

- direct cost to the National Health Service (NHS)
- indirect cost to society
- personal impact of PD on individuals with the condition and their family and carers.

The direct costs of treatment to the NHS have been estimated at approximately £2,298 (£ 1998) per patient per year.[10] Significant cost drivers include the onset of motor fluctuations and dyskinesias.[11] The condition is a frequent cause of falls and thus fractures and even death.[12]

The total annual cost of care including NHS, social services and private expenditure per patient in the UK has been estimated at approximately £5,993 (£ 1998).[10] This results in direct costs of approximately £599,300,000 per year in the UK for 100,000 individuals with PD.[10]

Total costs of care increase with age and disease severity.[10] Costs to the NHS were approximately 38% of the total costs.[10]

1.4   How to use this guideline

The purpose of this guideline is to support clinical judgement, not to replace it. This means the treating clinician should:

- take into consideration any contraindications in deciding whether or not to administer any treatment recommended by this guideline
- consider the appropriateness of any recommended treatment for a particular patient in terms of the patient's relevant clinical and non-clinical characteristics.

Wherever possible, before administering any treatment the treating clinician should follow good practice in terms of:

- discussing with the patient why the treatment is being offered and what health outcomes are anticipated
- highlighting any possible adverse events or side-effects that have been associated with the treatment
- obtaining explicit consent to administer the treatment.

For those recommendations involving pharmacological treatment, the most recent edition of the British National Formulary (BNF) should be followed for the determination of:

- indications
- drug dosage
- method and route of administration
- contraindications
- supervision and monitoring
- product characteristics

except in those cases where guidance is provided within the recommendation itself.

2 Methodology

2.1 Aim

The aim of the National Collaborating Centre for Chronic Conditions (NCC-CC) is to provide a user-friendly, clinical evidence-based guideline for the NHS in England and Wales that:

- offers best clinical advice for PD
- is based on best published evidence and expert consensus
- takes into account patient choice and informed decision making
- defines the major components of NHS care provision for PD
- indicates areas suitable for clinical audit
- details areas of uncertainty or controversy requiring further research
- provides a choice of guideline versions for different audiences.

2.2 Scope

The guideline was developed in accordance with a scope, which detailed the remit of the guideline originating from the Department of Health and specified those aspects of PD to be included and excluded.

Prior to the commencement of the guideline development, the scope was subjected to stakeholder consultation in accordance with processes established by NICE.[1,13] The full scope is shown in Appendix A.

The guideline covers:

- diagnoses of PD and parkinsonism
- treatment of idiopathic PD.

The scope excludes:

- juvenile onset PD (in people younger than 20 years of age)
- treatment of parkinsonism (a neurological disorder that manifests with hypokinesia, tremor or muscular rigidity) and other tremulous disorders (for example, essential tremor).

The guideline is relevant to primary, secondary and tertiary NHS care settings.

2.3 Audience

The guideline is primarily intended to provide guidance for NHS staff, but will also have relevance to the following people or organisations:

- all healthcare professionals
- people with the disease and carers of these people
- patient support groups
- commissioning organisations
- service providers.

2.4 Involvement of people with Parkinson's disease

The NCC-CC was keen to ensure that the views and preferences of people with PD and their carers informed all stages of the guideline. This was achieved:

- by consulting the Patient Information Unit housed within NICE during the pre-development (scoping) and final validation stages of the guideline
- by having a person with PD and a user organisation representative on the Guideline Development Group (GDG).

The patient and/or a representative of the user organisation were present at every meeting of the GDG. They were involved at all stages of the guideline development process and were able to consult with their wider constituencies.

2.5 Guideline limitations

The limitations of the guideline are as follows:

- Clinical guidelines usually do not cover issues of service delivery, organisation or provision (unless specified in the remit from the Department of Health).
- NICE is primarily concerned with health services and so recommendations are not provided for social services and the voluntary sector. However, the guideline may address important issues in how NHS clinicians interface with these other sectors.
- Generally the guideline does not cover rare, complex, complicated or unusual conditions.

2.6 Other work relevant to the guideline

This guideline has been developed with the knowledge that other national work on PD and chronic neurological conditions has been completed or is in progress. This includes:

- the National Service Framework (NSF) for Long-term (Neurological) Conditions[14]
- the NSF for Older People[15]
- NICE Guideline on Falls[16]
- NICE Guideline on Dementia[17]
- NICE Guideline on Depression[18]
- NICE Guideline on Epilepsy[19]
- NICE Guidance on Alzheimer's Disease[20]
- NICE Guideline on Anxiety[21]
- NICE Guideline on Nutrition[22]
- NICE Guidance on Deep Brain Stimulation[23]

2.7 The process of guideline development

The development of this evidence-based clinical guideline draws upon the methods described by the NICE Guideline Development Methods manual[1,13] and the methodology pack specifically developed by the NCC-CC for each chronic condition guideline.[24] The developers' role and remit is summarised in Table 2.1.

Table 2.1 Role and remit of the developers	
National Collaborating Centre for Chronic Conditions (NCC-CC)	The NCC-CC was set up in 2001 and is housed within the Royal College of Physicians (RCP). The NCC-CC undertakes commissions received from the National Instiutute for Health and Clinical Excellence (NICE). A multi-professional partners' board inclusive of patient groups and NHS management governs the NCC-CC.
NCC-CC Technical Team	The Technical Team met and comprised the following members: GDG group leader GDG clinical advisor Information scientist Research fellow Project manager Health economist Administrative personnel.
Guideline Development Group (GDG)	The GDG met monthly for 13 months (2004 to 2006) and comprised a multidisciplinary team of professionals, service users (a person with PD), carers, and user organisation representatives who were supported by the Technical Team. The GDG membership details including patient representation and professional groups are detailed in the GDG Membership table at the front of this guideline.
Guideline Project Executive (PE)	The PE was involved in overseeing all phases of the guideline. It also reviewed the quality of the guideline and compliance with the Department of Health remit and NICE scope. The PE comprised: NCC-CC Director NCC-CC Manager NCC-CC Senior Research Fellow NICE Commissioning Manager Technical Team.
Sign-off workshop	At the end of the guideline development process the GDG met to review and agree all the guideline recommendations.

Members of the GDG declared any interests in accordance with the NICE technical manual.[1] A register is available from the NCC-CC: **ncc-cc@rcplondon.ac.uk**

The basic steps in the process of producing a guideline are:

- developing clinical evidence-based questions
- systematically searching for the evidence
- critically appraising the evidence
- incorporating health economics advice
- distilling and synthesising the evidence and writing recommendations
- grading the evidence statements and recommendations
- agreeing the recommendations
- structuring and writing the guideline
- updating the guideline.

▷ Developing evidence-based questions

The Technical Team drafted a series of clinical questions that covered the guideline scope. The GDG and Project Executive refined and approved these questions, which are shown in Appendix B.

▷ Searching for the evidence

The information scientist developed a search strategy for each clinical question. In addition, the health economist searched for supplemental papers to inform models. Key words for the search were identified by the GDG. Papers that were published or accepted for publication in peer-reviewed journals were considered as evidence by the GDG. Conference paper abstracts and non-English language papers were excluded from all searches.

Each clinical question dictated the appropriate study design that was prioritised in the search strategy, but the strategy was not limited solely to these study types. The research fellow or health economist identified titles and abstracts from the search results that appeared to be relevant to the question. Exclusion lists were generated for each question together with the rationale for the exclusion. The exclusion lists were presented to the GDG. Full papers were obtained where relevant. Literature search details are shown in Appendix B.

▷ Appraising the evidence

The research fellow or health economist, as appropriate, critically appraised the full papers. In general no formal contact was made with authors; however, there were ad hoc occasions when this was required in order to clarify specific details. Critical appraisal checklists were compiled for each full paper. One research fellow undertook the critical appraisal and data extraction. The evidence was considered carefully by the GDG for accuracy and completeness.

All procedures are fully compliant with the:
- NICE methodology as detailed in *Guideline development methods – information for National Collaborating Centres and guideline developers'* manual[1]
- NCC-CC quality assurance document and systematic review chart, available at **www.rcplondon.ac.uk/college/ceeu/ncccc_index.htm.**

▷ Incorporating health economics advice

Due to the appointment of the health economist midway through the guideline development, the areas for health economic evidence were considered after the formation of the clinical questions. The health economist reviewed the clinical questions to consider the potential application of health economic evidence. Five key areas were separately identified by the clinical lead.

After agreement and selection of specific areas, the information scientist performed a literature search using economic filters on the related clinical questions. No study design criteria were imposed *a priori*. The searches were not limited to randomised controlled trials (RCTs) or formal economic evaluations. See the earlier section on 'Searching for the evidence' for details of the systematic search by the information scientist. The health economist reviewed titles and abstracts identified in the economic searches, and full papers were obtained as appropriate. The health economist critically appraised the full papers and the relevant data were presented to the GDG at subsequent GDG meetings. See the previous section for information on critically appraising the evidence.

The health economist performed supplemental literature searches using key search terms in the York Centre for Review and Dissemination database, the NHS Economic Evaluation database, PubMed and the Google search engine to obtain additional information for modelling. Areas were modelled due to the limited amount of evidence in or relevance to the UK setting. Assumptions and designs of the models were explained and agreed by the GDG members during meetings and validated by an additional health economist.

▷ Distilling and synthesising the evidence and writing recommendations

The evidence from each full paper was distilled into an evidence table and synthesised into evidence statements before being presented to the GDG. This evidence was then reviewed by the GDG and used as a basis upon which to formulate recommendations.

Evidence tables are available at:
www.rcplondon.ac.uk/pubs/online_home.htm

▷ Agreeing the recommendations

The sign-off workshop employed formal consensus techniques to:
- ensure that the recommendations reflected the evidence base
- approve recommendations based on lesser evidence or extrapolations from other situations
- reach consensus recommendations where the evidence was inadequate
- debate areas of disagreement and finalise recommendations.

The sign-off workshop also reached agreement on the following:
- five to ten key priorities for implementation
- five key research recommendations
- algorithms.

In prioritising key recommendations for implementation, the sign-off workshop also took into account the following criteria:
- high clinical impact
- high impact on reducing variation
- more efficient use of NHS resources
- allowing the patient to reach critical points in the care pathway more quickly.

The audit criteria provide suggestions of areas for audit in line with the key recommendations for implementation.[2]

▷ Structuring and writing the guideline

The guideline is divided into sections for ease of reading. For each section the layout is similar and is described below.

Table 2.2 Grading the evidence statements and recommendations

Levels of evidence		Classification of recommendations	
Level	**Type of evidence**	**Class**	**Evidence**
1++	High-quality meta-analysis (MA), systematic reviews (SR) of randomised controlled trials (RCTs), or RCTs with a very low risk of bias	A	Level 1++ and directly applicable to the target population *or* Level 1+ and directly applicable to the target population **AND** consistency of results Evidence from NICE technology appraisal
1+	Well-conducted MA, SR or RCTs, or RCTs with a low risk of bias		
1−	MA, SR of RCTs, or RCTs with a high risk of bias	Not used as a basis for making a recommendation	
2++	High-quality SR of case-control or cohort studies High-quality case-control or cohort studies with a very low risk of confounding, bias or chance and a high probability that the relationship is causal	B	Level 2++, directly applicable to the target population and demonstrating overall consistency of results *or* Extrapolated evidence from 1++ or 1+
2+	Well-conducted case-control or cohort studies with a low risk of confounding, bias or chance and a moderate probability that the relationship is causal		
2−	Case-control or cohort studies with a high risk of confounding, bias or chance and a significant risk that the relationship is not causal	Not used as a basis for making a recommendation	
3	Non-analytic studies (for example case reports, case series)	C	Level 2+, directly applicable to the target population and demonstrating overall consistency of results *or* Extrapolated evidence from 2++
4	Expert opinion, formal consensus	D	Level 3 or 4 *or* Extrapolated from 2+ *or* Formal consensus
		D (GPP)	A good practice point (GPP) is a recommendation based on the experience of the GDG

Diagnostic study level of evidence and classification of recommendation was also included.[1]

- *Clinical introduction:* sets a succinct background and describes the clinical context.
- *Methodological introduction:* describes any issues or limitations that were apparent when reading the evidence base.
- *Evidence statements:* provide a synthesis of the evidence base and usually describe what the evidence showed in relation to the outcomes of interest.
- *Health economics:* presents, where appropriate, an overview of the cost-effectiveness evidence-base.
- *From evidence to recommendation:* sets out the GDG decision-making rationale and provides a clear and explicit audit trail from the evidence to the evolution of the recommendations.
- *Recommendations:* provides stand-alone, action-oriented recommendations.

▷ Evidence tables

The evidence tables are not published as part of the full guideline but are available on-line at **www.rcplondon.ac.uk/pubs/books/pd**. These describe comprehensive details of the primary evidence that was considered during the writing of each section.

▷ Writing the guideline

The first draft version of the guideline was drawn up by the Technical Team in accord with the decision of the GDG. The guideline was then submitted for two formal rounds of public and stakeholder consultation prior to publication.[1,13] The registered stakeholders for this guideline are detailed in Appendix I. Editorial responsibility for the full guideline rests with the GDG.

Table 2.3 Versions of this guideline	
Full version	Details the recommendations. The supporting evidence base and the expert considerations of the GDG. Available at **www.rcplondon.ac.uk/pubs/books/PD**
NICE version	Documents the recommendations without any supporting evidence. Available at **www.nice.org.uk/page.aspx?o=guidelines.completed**
Quick reference guide	An abridged version. Available at **www.nice.org.uk/page.aspx?o=guidelines.completed**
Information for the public	A lay version of the guideline recommendations. Available at **www.nice.org.uk/page.aspx?o=guidelines.completed**

▷ Updating the guideline

Literature searches were repeated for all of the evidence-based questions at the end of the GDG development process, allowing any relevant papers published up until February 2005 to be considered. Future guideline updates will consider evidence published after this cut-off date.

Two years after publication of the guideline, NICE will commission a National Collaborating Centre to determine whether the evidence base has progressed significantly to alter the guideline recommendations and warrant an early update. If not, the guideline will be updated approximately 4 years after publication.[1,13]

2.8 Disclaimer

Healthcare providers need to use clinical judgement, knowledge and expertise when deciding whether it is appropriate to apply guidelines. The recommendations cited here are a guide and may not be appropriate for use in all situations. The decision to adopt any of the recommendations cited here must be made by the practitioner in light of individual patient circumstances, the wishes of the patient, clinical expertise and resources.

The NCC-CC disclaims any responsibility for damages arising out of the use or non-use of these guidelines and the literature used in support of these guidelines.

2.9 Funding

The National Collaborating Centre for Chronic Conditions was commissioned by the National Institute for Health and Clinical Excellence to undertake the work on this guideline.

THE GUIDELINE

3 | Key messages

In this chapter three essential components of the guideline will be discussed:
- key recommendations for implementation
- audit criteria
- algorithm.

Recommendations for implementation consist of recommendations selected by the GDG that highlight the main areas likely to have the most significant impact on patient care and patient outcomes in the NHS as a whole.[1,13]

Audit criteria are explicit statements developed from the recommendations for implementation, used to define the structure of care, process or outcome that is to be measured.[1,13]

The algorithm is a flowchart of the clinical decision pathway described in the clinical chapters.[1,13]

Another important section of the guideline is Chapter 12, 'Research recommendations'. This chapter discusses the GDG selected, priority areas for future PD research. Specific research questions are stated, the proposed trial structure is described and an explanatory paragraph is provided. General research recommendations are also included in this chapter.

3.1 Key priorities for implementation

▷ Referral to expert for accurate diagnosis

People with suspected PD should be referred quickly* and untreated to a specialist with expertise in the differential diagnosis of this condition.

▷ Diagnosis and expert review

The diagnosis of PD should be reviewed regularly** and reconsidered if atypical clinical features develop.

Acute levodopa and apomorphine challenge tests should not be used in the differential diagnosis of parkinsonian syndromes.

▷ Regular access to specialist nursing care

People with PD should have regular access to the following:
- clinical monitoring and medication adjustment
- a continuing point of contact for support, including home visits, when appropriate

---

*The GDG considered that people with suspected mild PD should be seen within 6 weeks but new referrals in later disease with more complex problems require an appointment within 2 weeks.
**The GDG considered that people diagnosed with PD should be seen at regular intervals of 6 to 12 months to review their diagnosis.

- a reliable source of information about clinical and social matters of concern to people with PD and their carers,

which may be provided by a Parkinson's disease nurse specialist (PDNS).

▷ Access to physiotherapy

Physiotherapy should be available for people with PD. Particular consideration should be given to:
- gait re-education, improvement of balance and flexibility
- enhancement of aerobic capacity
- improvement of movement initiation
- improvement of functional independence, including mobility and activities of daily living
- provision of advice regarding safety in the home environment.

▷ Access to occupational therapy

Occupational therapy should be available for people with PD. Particular consideration should be given to:
- maintenance of work and family roles, employment, home care and leisure activities
- improvement and maintenance of transfers and mobility
- improvement of personal self-care activities such as eating, drinking, washing and dressing
- environmental issues to improve safety and motor function
- cognitive assessment and appropriate intervention.

▷ Access to speech and language therapy

Speech and language therapy should be available for people with PD. Particular consideration should be given to:
- improvement of vocal loudness and pitch range, including speech therapy programmes such as Lee Silverman Voice Treatment (LSVT)
- teaching strategies to optimise speech intelligibility
- ensuring an effective means of communication is maintained throughout the course of the disease, including use of assistive technologies
- review and management to support the safety and efficiency of swallowing and to minimise the risk of aspiration.

▷ Palliative care

Palliative care requirements of people with PD should be considered throughout all phases of the disease.

People with PD and their carers should be given the opportunity to discuss end-of-life issues with appropriate healthcare professionals.

3.2 Audit criteria

The audit criteria shown in Table 3.1 are linked to the key priorities for implementation (see previous section). These are intended to be suggestions to aid and monitor the implementation of this guideline at the level of an NHS trust or similar scale healthcare provider.

Table 3.1 Audit criteria

Recommendation	Audit criterion	Exceptions
Referral to expert for accurate diagnosis		
People with suspected PD should be referred quickly* and untreated to a specialist with expertise in the differential diagnosis of this condition. *In suspected mild PD people should be seen within 6 weeks, but new referrals in later disease with more complex problems require an appointment within 2 weeks.	100% of people with suspected PD are seen within 6 weeks of GP referral.	None
Diagnosis and expert review		
The diagnosis of PD should be reviewed regularly** and reconsidered if atypical features develop. **At 6–12-month intervals.	100% of people with PD are reviewed at 6–12 month intervals.	None
Acute levodopa and apomorphine challenge tests should not be used in the differential diagnosis of parkinsonian syndromes.	0% of people with suspected PD are offered acute levodopa and/or apomorphine challenge tests for the differential diagnosis of parkinsonian syndromes.	None
Regular access to specialist nursing care		
People with PD should have regular access to the following: • clinical monitoring and medication adjustment • a continuing point of contact for support, including home visits, when appropriate • a reliable source of information about clinical and social matters of concern to people with PD and their carers, which may be provided by a PDNS.	100% of people with PD have access to a PDNS or other professional capable of providing: • clinical monitoring and medication adjustment • a continuing point of contact for support, including home visits, when appropriate • a reliable source of information about clinical and social matters of concern to people with PD and their carers.	None
Access to physiotherapy		
Physiotherapy should be available for people with PD. Particular consideration should be given to: • gait re-education, improvement of balance and flexibility • enhancement of aerobic capacity • improvement of movement initiation • improvement of functional independence, including mobility and activities of daily living • provision of advice regarding safety in the home environment.	For 100% of people with PD, at diagnosis and each regular review, physiotherapy is available and appropriate referral is activated. This is recorded in the patient's notes.	None

continued

Table 3.1 Audit criteria – *continued*

Recommendation	Audit criterion	Exceptions
Access to occupational therapy		
Occupational therapy should be available for people with PD. Particular consideration should be given to: • maintenance of work and family roles, employment, home care and leisure activities • improvement and maintenance of transfers and mobility • improvement of personal self-care activities such as eating, drinking, washing and dressing • environmental issues to improve safety and motor function • cognitive assessment and appropriate intervention.	For 100% of people with PD, at diagnosis and each regular review, OT is available and appropriate referral is activated. This is recorded in the patient's notes.	None
Access to speech and language therapy		
Speech and language therapy should be available for people with PD. Particular consideration should be given to: • improvement of vocal loudness and pitch range, including speech therapy programmes such as Lee Silverman Voice Treatment (LSVT) • teaching strategies to optimise speech intelligibility • ensuring an effective means of communication is maintained throughout the course of the disease, including use of assistive technologies • review and management to support the safety and efficiency of swallowing and to minimise the risk of aspiration.	For 100% of people with PD, at diagnosis and each regular review, speech and language therapy is available and appropriate referral is activated. This is recorded in the patient's notes.	None
Palliative care		
Palliative care requirements of people with PD should be considered throughout all phases of the disease.	100% of people with PD should be given opportunities to discuss and ask questions about their palliative care requirements with appropriate healthcare professionals.	None

3.3 Parkinson's disease algorithm

Disease progression

| Diagnosis and early disease | Throughout disease | Later disease |

Interventions

Diagnosis and early disease

Refer untreated to a specialist who makes and reviews diagnosis:
- use UK PDS Brain Bank Criteria
- consider 123I-FP-CIT SPECT
- specialist should review diagnosis at regular intervals (6–12 months)

It is not possible to identify a universal first choice drug therapy for people with early PD. The choice of drug first prescribed should take into account:
- clinical and lifestyle characteristics
- patient preference

Throughout disease

Consider management of non-motor symptoms in particular:
- depression
- psychosis
- dementia
- sleep disturbance

Provide regular access to specialist care particularly for:
- clinical monitoring and medication adjustment
- a continuing point of contact for support, including home visits when appropriate, which may be provided by a Parkinson's disease nurse specialist

Consider access to rehabilitation therapies, particularly to:
- maintain independence, including activities of daily living and ensure home safety
- help balance, flexibility, gait, movement initiation
- enhance aerobic activity
- assess and manage communication and swallowing

Later disease

It is not possible to identify a universal first choice adjuvant drug therapy for people with later PD. The choice of drug prescribed should take into account:
- clinical and lifestyle characteristics
- patient preference

Consider apomorphine in people with severe motor complications unresponsive to oral medication:
- intermittent injections to reduce off time
- continuous subcutaneous infusion to reduce off time and dyskinesia

Consider surgery:
- bilateral STN stimulation for suitable people refractory to best medical therapy
- thalamic stimulation for people with severe tremor for whom STN stimulation is unsuitable

Communication

Reach collaborative care decisions by taking into account:
- patient preference and choice after provision of information
- clinical characteristics, patient lifestyle and interventions available

Provide communication and information about:
- PD services and entitlements
- falls, palliative care and end-of-life issues

Figure 3.1 Parkinson's disease algorithm: interventions for people with PD.

4 Communication with people with Parkinson's disease and their carers

'I'd like them to remember to ask the patient how he feels and to listen to the patient. I'd like them to be more aware that each patient is an individual.' (patient)[2]

'I think what would have really helped was if someone had encouraged me to keep asking questions. The more you find out the easier it is to understand.' (patient)[4]

4.1 Introduction

Good communication is at the heart of every interaction between people with PD, their carers and health professionals. Issues that need to be considered include:

- style, manner and frequency of communication
- content and means of transmission
- ease of access for those receiving information, and consistency of content
- recognition that people with PD have particular clinical problems requiring carefully and sensitively tailored communication
- communication goals including self-management by people with PD
- involvement of carers.

Communication for people with chronic diseases can be focused on two goals:

- collaborative care in which clinicians are seen as experts in medical conditions, while people with a condition are seen as experts in living with their own condition and are encouraged to identify their problems and define goals.
- self-management education that provides people with problem-solving and management skills for the self-care of a condition.

For people with PD the main objective should be collaborative care, although interventions such as the Expert Patient Programme,[25] which concentrates on self-management, will have a part to play for some individuals. In addition, the NSF for Long-term (Neurological) Conditions (2005),[14] especially Quality requirement 1, which relates to a person-centred service, should underpin the principles of communication with people with PD and their carers.

4.2 Methodology

Six studies[26–31] have addressed communication about the diagnosis of PD. Since there were few RCTs in this area, qualitative studies and cross-sectional studies using questionnaire data collection tools were included. The literature search included the area of self-help in relation to communication and education of people with PD. However, no studies were found which specifically addressed this topic.

Qualitative studies were assigned evidence level 3 in accordance with NICE guidance.[1]

A qualitative study[29,30] using an interpretive phenomenological method identified a number of themes, but did not include a clear audit trail demonstrating how these were derived from the original patient data collected.

A cross-sectional self-report questionnaire study[29,30] collected response data from physiotherapists and occupational therapists who observed video records of patients.

It should be noted that:

- the PROPATH program[26,27] was a pharmaceutically sponsored educational service only available in the USA
- the survey from the Parkinson's Disease Society (PDS)[31] was based on a questionnaire of members in the UK.

The PROPATH program consisted of a disease assessment questionnaire, which was completed by people with PD or their carer. The questionnaire was analysed and computer-generated reports were returned to physicians and individualised recommendation letters returned to people with PD. The questionnaires were analysed by an advisory board of neurologists with broad experience in movement disorders. The reports and recommendation letters were primarily aimed at reducing medication side effects.

4.3   Evidence statements

Two RCTs[26,27] were found, which assessed the effectiveness of the PROPATH education program, as a novel approach to communication with people with PD.

A 6-month follow-up PROPATH study[26] (N=155) showed multiple benefits of the PROPATH intervention which are listed in Table 4.1. (1+)

Table 4.1 Effectiveness of PROPATH program versus standard care	
Outcome measures (N=322)	**p value**
Rate of disease progression during the program*	0.03
Number of people with PD exercising	0.006
Medical utilisation (in terms of doctor visits)	0.06
Time 'off'	>0.01
Quality-of-life assessment: self-efficacy measure**	
6 months score	<0.05
Total score	<0.01

*Rate of disease progression was calculated by changes in summary score at particular times divided by elapsed time in years. The summary score was an average of on-score and off-score (from Unified Parkinson's Disease Rating Scale (UPDRS)), side-effects index, and patient global assessment.
**Self-efficacy was estimated by a battery of 15 questions, which were assessed on a 0 to 100 horizontal analogue scale.

A separate 12-month follow-up PROPATH study (N=73)[27] observed only one improved clinical outcome in the intervention group: 'patient perception of general health and psychological well-being', which declined in the standard care group (p=0.04). (1+)

A multinational Global Parkinson's Disease Survey[28] of people with PD (N=201) and their carers (N=176) assessed what factors affect health-related quality-of-life (HRQL). This study found three factors which had an impact on quality of life and explained 60% of the variability in HRQL between people with PD:
- depression as measured by the Beck Depression Inventory (BDI) (p<0.001)
- 'satisfaction with explanation of condition at diagnosis' (p<0.05)
- 'feelings of optimism' which may be related to the style and manner of communication, especially at initial diagnosis (p<0.05). (3)

An interpretative phenomenological study[29] in 16 people with PD identified the theme of 'gaining formal knowledge' and provided the following information on their perspectives:
- Once diagnosed, people with PD identified a need to know more about the condition.
- Information provided at diagnosis was difficult to process by most participants.
- By their own descriptions, they were in 'shock' and did not recall the dialogue between themselves and the diagnosing physicians.
- There were a few exceptions to this and some clearly recalled being given a diagnosis but very little additional information.
- The human significance was passed over and objectified by what is known about the disease and treatment. Self-care and day-to-day coping with the illness were ignored. (3)

In a questionnaire study,[30] physiotherapists and occupational therapists (N=91) were asked to compare the video-recorded conversations of people with PD (N=4) and people with cardiac conditions (N=4) without the soundtrack. The aim was for the therapists to gauge their initial impressions of the people seen. The therapists were told the people being interviewed suffered from a neurological disorder, but the clinical diagnosis was not revealed. The video-recorded conversations were of interviews conducted by two doctors each of whom conversed with two individuals from each group using a semi-structured script covering non-medical aspects of the their personal histories. The study found there were significant differences in the ratings for all 15 variables. The therapists observed the people with PD to be:
- more anxious/worried/apprehensive; angry/irritable/hostile; suspicious/unforthcoming; morose/sad/down; bored/detached; tense/ill at ease (p<0.001)
- more introverted/shy; anxious/dissatisfied; sensitive/emotional; passive/dependent; less intelligent (p<0.001)
- enjoying the conversation less well (p<0.001)
- relating less well to the interviewer (p<0.001)
- holding up their own end of the conversation less well (p<0.001). (3)

In addition to their observations, the therapists were asked how likeable the person with PD appeared to them. People with PD appeared less likeable (p<0.001). (3)

It is worth noting that the people with PD in the above study had mild to moderate symptoms and were leading active lives. The impressions made by the therapists were formed from a short exposure to them on a video recording and therefore have the potential of being modified by further contact and greater knowledge of the individual. These results indicate that negative impressions may be induced in clinicians by a lack of verbal expressiveness from the person with PD, and this could influence the development of their relationship with their clinician.

Another study[32] (N=1200) assessed patient satisfaction with the educational information they had received (it did not assess the amount of information provided or who provided it). The findings are summmarized as follows.

- The average patient education score indicated that participants were neither particularly satisfied nor dissatisfied with the information they received.
- There was no relation between this score and sex, age or Hoehn and Yahr stage.
- When the analysis included all patients, a higher patient education score was associated with higher HRQL scores in all subscales of the Short Form 36 (SF-36), except for physical function and bodily pain.
- Patients were most satisfied with regard to 'role emotional' and least satisfied with regard to 'general health.'
- After excluding patients with advanced disease (Hoehn and Yahr 4–5), the regression coefficient increased in several subscales (ie patients with less severe disease had better quality-of-life scores), see Table 4.2 for details.
- Scores in all subscales of SF-36 were generally lower in patients with more advanced disease, demonstrating that the disease stage is associated with a decline in HRQL involving all aspects of daily living.
- Motor complications associated with therapy had a substantial affect on each subscale of SF-36. (3)

Table 4.2 Relationship of patient education with SF-36 (regression coefficients of patient education score)

	All patients	Excluding Hoehn and Yahr (stage 4 and 5)
Physical functioning	–0.76	–0.47
Role – physical	3.74*	5.23*
Bodily pain	2.01	0.06
General health	2.10*	1.99
Vitality	3.32*	3.66*
Social functioning	3.04*	4.40*
Role – emotional	4.18*	4.91*
Mental health	2.83*	4.10*

Adjusted for age, sex, number of comorbidities, activities of daily living score, and complications of therapy. The patient education score was 1 for 'not at all satisfied' and 5 for 'very satisfied' with information given. Therefore the difference in subscale score of SF-36 between two extremes was fourfold the number in the table.
*p<0.05.

The UK PDS[31] questioned 2,500 of their members from November 1997 to January 1998, regarding communication. Of these members, 1,693 (68%) replied and details of selected responses are given in Table 4.3. (3)

Table 4.3 PDS survey (1999)[31]

Whether the person had PD explained to them on diagnosis (N=1,127)

	(%)
Very clearly explained	20
Fairly clearly explained	24
Neither clearly nor unclearly explained	9
Not very clearly explained	17
Not at all clearly explained	9
No explanation given	15

Whether people were given an opportunity to ask questions on diagnosis

Adequate opportunity	28
Fairly adequate opportunity	22
No opportunity at all	15
Did not want/feel able to ask questions at the time	22

How useful people find PD information resources (N=1,693)

	Very useful	Not very useful	Not used/ not available	Did not answer
Hospital doctor/consultant	56	19	14	12
PDS – local branch	40	7	36	17
GP	39	37	13	11
PDS – national office	36	9	36	19
People who have PD or care for someone with PD	36	7	36	21
Newspapers or magazines	32	24	26	19
Pharmacist	25	11	45	19
PDNS	24	3	56	17
Physiotherapist	23	9	50	18
Occupational therapist	19	7	56	19
Television/radio	19	29	32	20
Social services department	18	12	51	18
Speech therapist	16	7	58	19
PDS – field staff (eg area officer)	15	6	57	21

continued

Table 4.3 PDS survey (1999)[31] – continued

Subjects on which people need information (N=945)	(%)
New treatments that may be available in future	90
What drugs are available and/or their side effects	84
Specific health problems related to PD	81
How the disease is likely to affect me or the person I care for in the future	75
Aids and equipment and how to get them	49
How PD can affect personal relationships	44
How to get health or social services assistance	41
How to get welfare benefits and financial help	39
How to deal with difficulties in getting services for people with PD from insurance companies, banks, etc.	30
How to find a suitable holiday	29
How to find suitable respite care	26

4.4 From evidence to recommendation

People with PD have to live with the consequences of any clinical decision. Given the nature of the therapies currently available for the condition, there are difficult trade-offs to be made over time between the beneficial therapeutic effects and the short- and long-term adverse consequences of a particular treatment. The choice of initial therapy should aim to optimise the quality of life over the whole expected lifespan of an individual. It is essential that these decisions are specific to an individual and agreed between the person with PD and the appropriate clinicians after a period of reflection including involvement of the family.

The evidence shows that the way in which the diagnosis of PD is communicated is important and often not well done. People with PD may need the information originally given at diagnosis to be repeated and will want more information as the condition progresses. This is one important role that could be carried out by a health professional such as the PDNS (see Chapter 10). No evidence is available on what format this information should best be given in, but a range of products are already available from the UK PDS.

Particular features that need to be taken into account when communicating with people with PD are:
- occurrence of cognitive impairment and depression
- occurrence of a communication impairment (which increases in severity with increasing severity of the disease process)
- negative impression that may be given by a person with PD
- need for emotional support
- involvement of carers.

Effective communication requires well-trained staff and an environment that enables sensitive discussions, as these discussions might lead to emotional distress. The UK PDS recently published guidance about communication with people with PD and their carers.[33] The recommendations arose from a group of 17 people with PD, with ages ranging from 47 to 67, and their carers. The document is shown in Appendix C.

It is important to communicate with carers, particularly when people with PD have cognitive impairment or depression. Carers need:

- general factual information about the condition
- specific information, if permission is given, about the person with PD
- information about services and entitlements to care assessment and support procedures
- advice and support both to optimise the quality of the communication interaction and also to continue effective communication with the person with PD as the condition progresses
- advice and support to maintain their health and well-being.

RECOMMENDATIONS

R1 Communication with people with PD should be aimed towards empowering them to participate in the judgements and choices about their own care. **D**

R2 Discussions should be aimed at achieving a balance between the provision of honest, realistic information about the condition and the promotion of a feeling of optimism. **D**

R3 Because people with PD may develop impaired cognitive ability, a communication deficit and/or depression, they should be provided with:

- both oral and written communication throughout the course of the disease, which should be individually tailored and reinforced as necessary
- consistent communication from the professionals involved. **D (GPP)**

R4 Families and carers should be given information about the condition, their entitlements to care assessment and the support services available. **D (GPP)**

R5 People with PD should have a comprehensive care plan agreed between the individual, their family and/or carers and specialist and secondary healthcare providers. **D (GPP)**

R6 People with PD should be offered an accessible point of contact with specialist services. This could be provided by a Parkinson's disease nurse specialist. **D (GPP)**

R7 All people with PD who drive should be advised to inform the Driver and Vehicle Licensing Agency (DVLA) and their car insurer of their condition at the time of diagnosis. **D (GPP)**

5 | Diagnosing Parkinson's disease

*'It knocked me for six . . . I became very low . . . I thought it can't
be me . . . it's just elderly people who got it.'* (patient)[2]

*'I found it hard to cope with life . . . I didn't tell anyone . . .
I couldn't face the reality of it.'* (patient)[2]

5.1 Definition and differential diagnosis

There are many manifestations of PD but the classical diagnostic symptoms are:

* slowness and poverty of movement
* stiffness
* shaking.

The physical signs of PD include:

* slowness of movement (bradykinesia)
* poverty of movement (hypokinesia), eg loss of facial expression and arm swing, difficulty with fine movements
* rigidity
* rest tremor.

At diagnosis, these signs are usually unilateral, but they become bilateral as the disease progresses. Later in the disease additional signs may be present including postural instability (eg tendency to fall backwards after a sharp pull from the examiner: the 'pull test'), cognitive impairment and orthostatic hypotension (OH).

There is no single way to define Parkinson's disease or what is often called idiopathic Parkinson's disease in order to differentiate it from other causes of parkinsonism, such as multiple system atrophy (MSA) and progressive supranuclear palsy (PSP).

PD is traditionally defined, pathologically, by the finding of Lewy bodies and degeneration of catecholaminergic neurones at post-mortem. Using a pathological definition of PD is problematic for a number of reasons:

* A pathological diagnosis is not practical in life.
* Lewy body inclusions in catecholaminergic neurones are seen in individuals without clinical evidence of PD; it is presumed that these are pre-clinical cases.
* Lewy bodies have not been found in otherwise typical individuals with PD with Parkin mutations, although such rare young-onset genetic cases of PD might be said not to have idiopathic PD.

In recent years, attempts to define PD genetically have become possible with the discovery of monogenic forms of the disease. However, such families account for a very small proportion of cases.

Another potential way to diagnose PD is using the response to dopaminergic medication. However, this dopaminergic responsiveness can be seen in conditions other than PD such as MSA.

The decline in dopaminergic neurones identified by radionuclide positron emission tomography (PET) or single photon emission computed tomography (SPECT) has also been proposed as a method of defining PD. Unfortunately, this decline is seen in conditions other than PD such as MSA and PSP.

Given these difficulties, it is generally accepted that the diagnosis of PD should be based on clinical findings. The most widely accepted clinical criteria for the diagnosis of PD are those introduced by the UK PDS Brain Bank Criteria (Table 5.1).[35]

It is important to make an accurate diagnosis in a person with suspected PD as this has an important bearing on prognosis. People with PD will have a longer life expectancy than those with MSA or PSP and will respond better to dopaminergic medication.

PD must also be differentiated from other conditions presenting with tremor (Table 5.2). This can be particularly difficult as PD can present with a postural and action tremor similar to that seen in essential tremor.

In addition, PD must be differentiated from other causes of a parkinsonian syndrome or parkinsonism (Table 5.3). The most common problems arise with multiple cerebral infarction and degenerative parkinsonian syndromes such as MSA and PSP. Differential diagnosis can also be difficult in elderly people since extrapyramidal symptoms and signs are common.[34]

Table 5.1 UK PDS Brain Bank Criteria for the diagnosis of PD[35]

Step 1. Diagnosis of a parkinsonian syndrome

Bradykinesia and at least one of the following:
- muscular rigidity
- rest tremor (4–6 Hz)
- postural instability unrelated to primary visual, cerebellar, vestibular or proprioceptive dysfunction.

Step 2. Exclusion criteria for PD

History of:
- repeated strokes with stepwise progression
- repeated head injury
- antipsychotic or dopamine-depleting drugs
- definite encephalitis and/or oculogyric crises on no drug treatment
- more than one affected relative
- sustained remission
- negative response to large doses of levodopa (if malabsorption excluded)
- strictly unilateral features after 3 years
- other neurological features: supranuclear gaze palsy, cerebellar signs, early severe autonomic involvement, Babinski sign, early severe dementia with disturbances of language, memory or praxis
- exposure to known neurotoxin
- presence of cerebral tumour or communicating hydrocephalus on neuroimaging.

Step 3. Supportive criteria for PD

Three or more required for diagnosis of definite PD:
- unilateral onset
- rest tremor present
- progressive disorder
- persistent asymmetry affecting the side of onset most
- excellent response to levodopa
- severe levodopa-induced chorea
- levodopa response for over 5 years
- clinical course of over 10 years.

Table 5.2 Common causes of tremor
Rest tremor
Parkinson's disease
Postural and action tremor
Essential tremor
Exaggerated physiological tremor
Hyperthyroidism
Drug-induced (eg β-agonists)
Dystonic tremor
Intention tremor
Cerebellar disorders

Table 5.3 Causes of a parkinsonian syndrome
Parkinson's disease
Alzheimer's disease
Multiple cerebral infarction
Drug-induced parkinsonism (eg phenothiazines)
Other degenerative parkinsonian syndromes:
• progressive supranuclear palsy (Steele–Richardson–Olszewski syndrome)
• multiple system atrophy (previously Shy–Drager syndrome, olivopontocerebellar atrophy and striatonigral degeneration)

RECOMMENDATION

R8   PD should be suspected in people presenting with tremor, stiffness, slowness, balance problems and/or gait disorders.   **D (GPP)**

5.1.1 Methodological limitations of the diagnostic studies

When interpreting the literature about PD diagnosis, the following methodological issues should be considered:

- lack of long-term prospective clinical and pathological follow-up as a reference standard
- lack of operational definitions such as defining specialists or clinical diagnostic criteria
- unclear whether investigators were blinded to initial diagnosis
- sample sizes necessarily limited by the number of cases available with neuropathological outcomes
- PD trial age groups are often young as studies were performed by neurologists who see a younger population of people with PD
- most studies included people with established disease lasting some years
- varying geographical locations

- some studies are in specialised units and may not reflect the diagnostic accuracy of other units in the UK
- exclusion of some studies using magnetic resonance volumetry and magnetic resonance spectroscopy (MRS) as they lacked appropriate population, intervention and outcome criteria
- lack of statistical details of diagnostic accuracy such as sensitivity, specificity and positive predictive values
- lack of economic evaluations of SPECT.

5.2 Clinical versus post-mortem diagnosis

Most experienced specialists have adopted the UK PDS Brain Bank Clinical Criteria (Table 5.1) for the diagnosis of PD.

How do these compare with the accuracy of pathological diagnosis?

5.2.1 Methodology

Three diagnostic studies were found that assessed the accuracy of clinical diagnosis in parkinsonism compared with autopsy.[36–38] These studies compared clinical diagnosis, at various stages of disease progression, to a final diagnosis including details of autopsy findings. The clinical diagnosis was determined using the UK PDS Brain Bank Criteria (Table 5.1) in two of three studies.[37,38] A third study determined a diagnosis of PD when at least two of the three cardinal signs (bradykinesia, rigidity and resting tremor) were present.[36]

5.2.2 Evidence statements

Two studies (N=59[36] and N=100[37]) examined people with a terminal diagnosis of PD and found the frequency of people misdiagnosed with PD (ie they did not meet the pathological criteria at post-mortem) was 35% and 24% respectively.[36,37] When recommended diagnostic criteria (UK PDS Brain Bank) were retrospectively applied, diagnostic accuracy increased from 70% to 82%.[37] (DS II)

A more recent UK PDS Brain Bank study[38] examined the brains of 143 people with parkinsonism. These people had previously been seen by a neurologist, with five dedicated movement disorder specialists seeing 92% of the cases, and been given a clinical diagnosis of PD or alternative parkinsonian condition. The clinical diagnosis was later revised in 44 of 122 cases where full follow-up information was available after a mean of 3.4 (range 0.5–12) years. The sensitivity of the final PD clinical diagnosis was 91%, a specificity of 98% and a positive predictive value of 99% (72 out of 73 correctly diagnosed). (DS II)

5.2.3   From evidence to recommendation

The pathological studies emphasise the need for particular care in making a clinical diagnosis of PD. There is limited evidence to suggest that the UK PDS Brain Bank Criteria have adequate sensitivity and specificity in comparison with post-mortem findings. The accuracy of diagnosis using the Brain Bank criteria increases as the condition progresses.

The availability of PD brain tissue has fostered much valuable research in recent years and should be encouraged in the future. Diagnostic information derived from post-mortem examination can also be of value to the families of individual patients.

RECOMMENDATIONS

R9   PD should be diagnosed clinically and based on the UK Parkinson's Disease Society Brain
Bank Criteria.   **B (DS)**

R10   Clinicians should be encouraged to discuss with patients the possibility of tissue
donation to a brain bank for purposes of diagnostic confirmation and research.   **D (GPP)**

5.3   Expert versus non-expert diagnosis

The diagnosis of PD could be made in primary care by the person's GP or in secondary care by a neurologist, geriatrician or general physician. More recently, PDNSs and other health professionals are developing diagnostic skills. Each may have different levels of expertise in evaluating people with possible PD.

What is the evidence that someone with special expertise is more accurate in diagnosing PD than someone with little experience?

5.3.1   Methodology

Four diagnostic studies[39–42] were found looking at the accuracy of PD diagnosis in a community-based population. The specialist diagnosis was based on the UK PDS Brain Bank criteria in four of the studies.[39,40,42] In one study[41] the expert diagnosis was based on the investigator's confidence in the diagnosis of PD, presence of atypical features, findings of imaging studies, response to levodopa and results of autopsy examinations. The criteria for the initial diagnoses were not specified in any of the trials. These studies were also performed on prevalent rather than incident PD populations.

5.3.2   Evidence statements

One study[39] (N=126) assessed the diagnostic accuracy of neurologist and geriatrician clinical expert diagnosis versus existing clinical diagnosis of parkinsonism from medical records by a non-expert clinician. The standard for comparison was diagnosis according to strict clinical diagnostic criteria (the UK PDS Brain Bank Criteria) after a detailed neurological interview and examination. The study found that neurologists and geriatricians had a sensitivity of 93.5% (95% CI 86.3 to 97.6) and specificity of 64.5% (95% CI 45.4 to 80.8) compared with 'non-specialist' sensitivity of 73.5% (95% CI 55.6 to 87.1) and specificity of 79.1% (95% CI 64.0 to 90.0) for diagnostic accuracy. While the positive predictive value of specialists was greater than for other doctors, negative predictive values were equivalent. (DS II)

Another study[40] applied the UK PDS Brain Bank criteria to 402 cases derived from a computerised list of people with PD receiving anti-parkinsonian medication from 74 general practices in North Wales. In 59% of cases, the GP made the initial diagnosis of PD. The people with PD were seen either at home or in a specialist movement disorder clinic where a neurological examination was performed. A definite PD diagnosis was made in 53% of all cases, thus the error rate in the community-ascertained cases was 47%. (DS II)

DATATOP (Deprenyl and Tocopherol Antioxidative Therapy of Parkinsonism) was a large, multi-site clinical trial[41] in the USA and Canada involving 800 people with early-stage PD who were cared for by 34 investigators with a major interest in movement disorders. A secondary analysis examined the number of people with PD with a change in diagnosis after a mean follow-up of 6 years. The study showed that only 8% had a revised diagnosis. The revised diagnosis was clinical and not based on strict criteria or pathology. (DS II)

The UK-PDRG study,[42] which investigated the long-term effectiveness of bromocriptine, selegiline and levodopa therapy, found a total of 49/782 people with PD (6%) had their diagnosis changed during the course of the trial. Individuals were eligible for inclusion in the study if they fulfilled criteria for a clinical diagnosis of PD. The authors do not state whether the revised diagnosis was made by one of the specialists performing the study, although this is likely. The authors also do not state whether a specialist or non-specialist conducted the initial diagnostic examination. (DS II)

5.3.3 From evidence to recommendation

These studies provide only circumstantial evidence on the diagnostic ability of experts versus non-experts. However, they show that the diagnosis of PD is wrong in around 47% of community-ascertained cases, 25% of non-expert secondary care diagnosed cases, and 6–8% of cases diagnosed by an expert in movement disorders.

Since medication can mask the symptoms and signs of PD, the GDG felt that people with suspected PD should be referred before treatment is commenced. This can be achieved only if people are seen quickly by experts, for an accurate diagnosis and commencement of treatment, if necessary.

The GDG also had experience that delay in making an accurate diagnosis can lead to psychological stress for the patient and their carer. Similarly, the need to revise an incorrect diagnosis that has, initially, been made by a non-expert can be stressful for patients.

The GDG acknowledges the timeline that the Department of Health and NHS are currently working towards for completion of diagnosis and treatment (18-week target). However, the GDG felt that in the case of PD it should not necessarily mean that patients would have to 'start' treatment within 18 weeks from GP referral but rather that this was when a 'treatment decision' was made for initial consultation and diagnosis.

RECOMMENDATION

R11   People with suspected PD should be referred quickly* and untreated to a specialist with expertise in the differential diagnosis of this condition.   **B (DS)**

5.4   Review of diagnosis

Given the error rate in making a diagnosis of PD, even in expert hands, it is apparent that the diagnosis should be kept under regular review.

What is the most appropriate frequency of follow-up after an initial diagnosis of PD?

5.4.1   Methodology

No trials were found which addressed the most appropriate frequency of follow-up of people with PD.

5.4.2   Evidence statements

No evidence was found on the most appropriate frequency of follow-up after the initial diagnosis of the disease.

5.4.3   From evidence to recommendation

In the absence of any evidence on the issue of frequency of follow-up, the GDG concluded that this should be based on clinical priority. In people with early mild symptoms of PD who may not even be on treatment yet, follow-up to check on the diagnosis and the need for treatment may be infrequent (every 6–12 months). Once treatment is commenced, follow-up may need to be more frequent (every 2–3 months) to assess the response to medication, titrate dosage and re-visit the diagnosis. In later disease, people with PD have more complex problems which require changes in medication. This may require review at frequent intervals (every 2–3 months).

RECOMMENDATION

R12   The diagnosis of PD should be reviewed regularly** and reconsidered if atypical clinical features develop.   **D (DS)**

---

*The GDG considered that people with suspected mild PD should be seen within 6 weeks, but new referrals in later disease with more complex problems require an appointment within 2 weeks.
**The GDG considered that people diagnosed with PD should be seen at regular intervals of 6–12 months to review their diagnosis.

5.5 Single photon emission computed tomography

In single photon emission computed tomography (SPECT), a gamma ray-emitting radioactive isotope is tagged to a molecule of interest (a tracer), which is given to the person with PD by intravenous injection. The labelled cocaine derivatives ^{123}I-β-CIT and ^{123}I-FP-CIT (N-ω-fluoropropyl-2β-carboxymethoxy-3β-(4-iodophenyl)tropane) have most commonly been used, although only the latter is licensed in the UK. These label the presynaptic dopamine re-uptake site and thus the presynaptic neurone, which can be visualised in two-dimensional images. These demonstrate normal uptake in the caudate and putamen in controls and in people with essential tremor, neuroleptic-induced parkinsonism or psychogenic parkinsonism, but reduced uptake in those with PD, PD with dementia, MSA or PSP.

How useful is SPECT in discriminating PD from alternative conditions?

5.5.1 Methodology

Fifteen studies addressed the diagnostic accuracy of SPECT scanning.[43–58] The reference standard was clinical diagnosis: eight out of the 16 studies[43,45–51] used the UK PDS Brain Bank Criteria, five studies[44,52–55] used 'established' clinical criteria and three studies[56–58] did not state the clinical criteria used to determine the diagnosis. Although many tracers are listed in the evidence statements, only ^{123}I-FP-CIT is licensed for use in the UK. The ^{123}I-β-CIT studies were included as it has a similar structure and labels the same receptors as the ^{123}I-FP-CIT tracer. The GDG agreed that this evidence is supportive of ^{123}I-FP-CIT studies and provides a consistency of effect.

5.5.2 Health economic methodology

Only one study met quality criteria that addressed the economic evaluation of SPECT.[59] This study was based on ^{123}I-FP-CIT SPECT effectiveness data, specificity and sensitivity of clinical examination and prevalence of PD were based predominantly on UK data. However, costs were based on German 2002 data.[59]

5.5.3 Evidence statements

For the differentiation of people with parkinsonism (ie PD, MSA or PSP) from people with essential tremor or controls using SPECT, all studies produced a high sensitivity (range 87% to 98.3%) and specificity (range 80% to 100%).[43,45,49,52,53] A summary of the evidence produced in these five studies is provided in Table 5.4 and Table 5.5. (DS Ib)

Three studies (N=80,[47,48,54] N=17,[47,48,54] N=183[47,48,54]) attempting to differentiate PD from other parkinsonian conditions (eg MSA, PSP) had insufficiently high levels of sensitivity (range 77% to 97%) and specificity (range 75% to 83%).[47,48,54] (DS Ib)

One study[58] found, by comparing the ^{123}I-β-CIT SPECT imaging diagnosis for people with parkinsonian syndrome with a clinical diagnosis (based on 6 months' follow-up), that there was disagreement between only three out of 35 cases (8.6%) with visual diagnosis and two out of 35 cases (5.7%) with quantitative imaging diagnosis. (DS Ib)

Table 5.4 Diagnostic accuracy of SPECT imaging: differentiation of tremulous disorders

Test	Number of participants		Sensitivity (%)	Specificity (%)	Grade
^{123}I-FP-CIT SPECT (institutional read)[45]	158 PD	27 ET	97	100	Ib
^{123}I-FP-CIT SPECT (consensus read)[45]	Same as above		95	93	Ib
^{123}I-FP-CIT SPECT[43]	38 PD	38 Non-PD	87	–	Ib
^{123}I-β-CIT SPECT [49]	60 PD and PSP	36 ET and controls	98	83	Ib
^{123}I-β-CIT SPECT: Striatum/cerebellum and putamen/ cerebellum binding ratio factors[52]	29 PD	62 controls and ET	98.3	–	Ib
	29 PD	32 ET	96.7		
^{123}I-β-CIT SPECT: Visual imaging analysis[58] Visual imaging analysis[58]	35 suspect PD		96	80	Ib
^{123}I-β-CIT SPECT: Quantitative imaging analysis[58]	Same as above		90	100	Ib

Institutional read = visual assessment of ^{123}I-FP-CIT striatal uptake by investigator blinded to clinical diagnosis. Consensus read = hard-copy images – agreement from three or more of the five panel members.
PD = parkinsonian syndrome; PSP = progressive supranuclear palsy; ET = essential tremor.

Table 5.5 Diagnostic accuracy of SPECT imaging: differentiation of PD and controls

Test	Number of participants		Sensitivity (%)	Specificity (%)	Grade
	PD	Controls			
^{123}I-β-CIT SPECT: Striatum/cerebellum binding ratio alone[52]	29	32	94.9	–	Ib
^{123}I-FP-CIT SPECT: Binding index in putamen contralateral to initially clinically affected side[50]	76	20	95	86	II
TRODAT-1 SPECT: Binding index in putamen contralateral to initially clinically affected side[50]	Same as above		92	70	II
TRODAT-1 SPECT: Logistic discriminant parametric mapping[53]	42	23	100	95	II
TRODAT-1 SPECT: Visual inspection[55]	188	45	98	86	Ib
TRODAT-1 SPECT: Quantitative analysis[55]	Same as above		98	88	Ib
TRODAT-1 SPECT: Contralateral putamen/occipital and contralateral putamen/caudate[57]	78	40	100	100	II
TRODAT-1 SPECT: Quantitative imaging analysis. Mean uptake in ipsilateral and contralateral posterior putamen[51]	29	38	0.79	0.92	II

TRODAT-1 = selective dopamine transporter technetium-99m labelled.
Logistic discriminant parametric mapping = technique to distinguish sets of data with maximum accuracy.

5.5.4 Health economic evidence statements

The economic findings indicated:[59]

- SPECT has greater sensitivity but costs more than clinical examination
- SPECT should not be used in all people with PD in place of initial clinical examination
- SPECT could be used to avoid the costs of treating people who do not suffer from PD.

For approximately an additional €733 in Euro 2002 (approximately £511), for the equivalent of a patient-month with adequate treatment, SPECT could be used to confirm a PD diagnosis in people with a positive clinical examination before the initiation of treatment.[59] Adequate treatment month equivalents (ATME) were used to reflect both duration of adequate treatment and severity of incorrect treatments. The authors indicated that a 0.55 ATME gain per patient is equivalent to approximately 17 additional days of treatment to a PD patient or withholding approximately 2 days of treatment and side effects to a patient who does not have PD.

The specificity of clinical examination and frequency of PD in the clinic population of PD had the greatest relative impact on the incremental cost-effectiveness ratio (ICER) of SPECT following positive clinical examination compared with clinical examination alone. In the sensitivity analysis, when the specificity of clinical examination is reduced to 0.80 (from 0.984) the ICER drops to €63 (approximately £44).[59] This suggests that as more non-PD cases are incorrectly classified as PD cases in clinical examination, the greater the cost-effectiveness of SPECT. When the frequency of PD in the clinic population is increased to 74% (from 53%) the ICER increases to €2,411 (approximately £1,697).[59] This suggests that the cost-effectiveness of SPECT decreases when the frequency of PD in the clinic population increases. In these populations, there may be fewer false-negative results and therefore fewer people incorrectly being treated for PD. This would mean there are fewer cost-savings from withholding incorrect treatment and therefore an increase in the relative cost-effectiveness of SPECT.

5.5.5 From evidence to recommendation

Considerable evidence supports the use of ^{123}I-FP-CIT SPECT in people with postural and/or action tremor of the upper limbs in the differentiation of essential tremor from a dopaminergic deficiency state. ^{123}I-FP-CIT SPECT cannot, with high accuracy, differentiate PD from other dopaminergic deficiency states such as MSA and PSP. Future work may demonstrate the value of this technique in differentiating parkinsonism due to neuroleptic medication and psychogenic parkinsonism from a dopaminergic deficiency state.

Several clinical trials using SPECT or PET to follow the progression of PD found that 4%,[60] 11%[61] and 14%[62] with a clinical diagnosis of PD had normal imaging at the start of the trial. Further long-term clinical follow-up of these people is required.

Due to the subjectivity of the effectiveness measurement, the GDG decided the economic study[59] does not support or refute the clinical recommendations. Further development of comparable effectiveness outcomes in diagnostic economic evaluations is required.

RECOMMENDATIONS

R13 ^{123}I-FP-CIT SPECT should be considered for people with tremor where essential tremor cannot be clinically differentiated from parkinsonism.   A (DS)

R14 ^{123}I-FP-CIT SPECT should be available to specialists with expertise in its use and interpretation.   D (DS)

5.6   Positron emission tomography

In positron emission tomography (PET), a positron-emitting radioactive isotope is tagged to a tracer molecule, which is administered by intravenous injection. The most frequently used positron-emitting isotope in this field is ^{18}fluorine, which is attached to dopa or deoxyglucose. ^{18}F-fluorodopa is taken up by the presynaptic dopaminergic neurones of the caudate and putamen (corpus striatum). ^{18}F-fluorodeoxyglucose (FDG) is taken up by all metabolically active cells and phosphorylated to a metabolite, which is trapped in the tissue for the time course of the study.

How valuable is PET in the differential diagnosis of parkinsonism?

5.6.1   Methodology

Six diagnostic studies[63–68] were found which addressed the effectiveness of PET scanning compared with clinical diagnosis in the differential diagnosis of a parkinsonian syndrome. No studies were found which compared the effectiveness of PET in the differentiation of PD from essential tremor.

5.6.2   Evidence statements

In one study[68] the diagnostic accuracy of ^{18}F-desmethoxy-fallypride PET imaging for the differential diagnosis of atypical (N=16) versus idiopathic (N=16) parkinsonian syndromes showed a threshold value of 2.495 (caudate uptake ratio). The sensitivity, specificity and accuracy were 74%, 100% and 86% respectively. Using this threshold, the positive and negative predictive values for the diagnosis of atypical parkinsonian syndromes were 100% and 76%. **(DS Ib)**

In one study[67] the multi-diagnosis group discriminate analysis from ^{18}F-FDG PET scan images found sensitivity of 75% and specificity of 100% in the PD group (N=8), sensitivity of 100% and specificity of 87% in the MSA group (N=9), and sensitivity of 86% and specificity of 94% in the PSP group (N=7). **(DS II)**

One study,[69] using ^{18}F-FDG uptake, reported 74% of all participants (early PD (N=15), atypical PD (N=9) and controls (N=15)) were correctly classified when regional cerebral glucose metabolism (rCMRGlc) was analysed. This diagnostic accuracy increased to 95% using topographical profile rating, which is a method for calculating participant scores for abnormal regional metabolic co-variance patterns in individual people with PD. **(DS II)**

One study (N=90),[63] using ^{18}F-fluorodopa uptake, found people with clinically diagnosed PD were correctly classified by PET in 64% of the cases and those with atypical parkinsonism (MSA or PSP) in 69% of the cases. **(DS II)**

In another study[70] the probability of the correct diagnosis by ^{18}F-fluorodopa PET was ≥99% for the majority of people with PD (40/41) and controls (26/28). **(DS II)**

5.6.3 From evidence to recommendation

PET has better spatial resolution than SPECT, so it might be anticipated that PET should be of value in differential diagnosis. However, the evidence for PET's role in differentiating PD from other parkinsonian conditions using FDG requires further confirmation. No work was found on PET's ability to differentiate PD from essential tremor. This lack of evidence stems from the high cost and poor availability of PET. Further research is required in this area.

RECOMMENDATIONS

R15   PET should not be used in the differential diagnosis of parkinsonian syndromes, except
in the context of clinical trials.   **B (DS)**

5.7   Magnetic resonance imaging

Structural magnetic resonance imaging (MRI) provides two- and three-dimensional images of intracranial structures using high magnetic field strengths to excite the hydrogen atoms in water molecules. In PD this technique has been used to examine various structures known to be involved in the pathology of the condition in the hope that it may prove of value in differential diagnosis.

How useful is structural MRI in the differential diagnosis of parkinsonian conditions and essential tremor?

5.7.1 Methodology

Eight diagnostic studies[64,66,71–76] were found which addressed the effectiveness of MRI compared with long-term clinical follow-up in diagnosing people with a parkinsonian syndrome. Various MRI scanning sequences were used.

5.7.2 Evidence statements

Seven of these studies[64,71–76] provided diagnostic accuracy data for MRI using various techniques. The results are summarised in Table 5.6.

Table 5.6 Diagnostic accuracy of MRI				
Technique	Participants (N)	Sensitivity (%)	Specificity (%)	Grade
Abnormal putaminal T2 hypointensity[71,72,74]	MSA-P (24) versus PD (27)	87.5	88.89	DS Ib
Proton density putaminal hyperintensity[71,72,74]	Same as above	83.3	100	
T1 MRI: midbrain superior profile[75,76]	PD (27) versus PSP (25)	68	88.8	
T1 MRI: midbrain atrophy[75,76]	Same as above	68	77.7	DS Ib
T2 MRI: tegmental hyperintensity[75,76]	Same as above	28	100	
Putaminal T2 hypointensity and T2 hyperintensity combined[73,74,76]	MSA (28) versus PD (32)	32	100	
Putaminal T2 hypointensity and T2 hyperintensity combined[73,74,76]	MSA (28) versus PSP (30)	32	93	
Putaminal T2 hypointensity and T2 hyperintensity combined[73,74,76]	MSA (28) versus CBD (26)	32	85	DS II
Overall MRI abnormalities[73,74,76]	PD (32) versus MSA (28)	71	91	
Overall MRI abnormalities[73,74,76]	PD (32) versus PSP (30)	70	91	
Overall MRI abnormalities[73,74,76]	PD (32) versus CBD (26)	92	91	
T1 MRI: voxel-based morphometry of cerebral peduncles and midbrain[74–76]	PSP (12) versus PD (12) and controls (12)	83	79	DS II
Diffusion-weighted MRI Putaminal rADC[64]	MSA-P (10) versus PD (11)	100	100	
Diffusion-weighted MRI Putaminal hyperintense rim[64]	Same as above	80	91	DS II
Diffusion-weighted MRI Putaminal atrophy[64]	Same as above	60	100	
Diffusion-weighted MRI Putaminal rADC[72,73,75]	PSP (10), PD (13) and MSA-P (12) versus clinical diagnosis	96	100	DS II

rADC = regional apparent diffusion coefficient; PSP = progressive supranuclear palsy; MSA-P = multiple system atrophy parkinsonian type; MSA-C = multiple system atrophy cerebellar type; CBD = corticobasalganglionic degeneration.

Another study[66] found non-concordance between neuroradiological diagnosis and clinical diagnosis in 2/21 people with PD, 5/14 people with MSA-P and 1/4 people with MSA-C. (DS II)

One study[75] reported only 15% of people with PD and 24% of those with PSP had abnormal T2 hypointensity in the posterolateral putamen and none had abnormal putaminal proton density hyperintensity. (DS Ib)

One study[74] found two false negatives in the PSP group (one had a diagnosis of clinically probable PSP and one clinically definite PSP) and five false positives (two were non-diseased controls and three had a diagnosis of PD). (DS II)

5.7.3 From evidence to recommendation

In expert hands structural MRI has proved of some value in differentiating PD from other types of parkinsonism, but further research is required before it can be recommended in routine clinical practice.

RECOMMENDATIONS

R16   Structural MRI should not be used in the differential diagnosis of PD.   B (DS)

R17   Structural MRI may be considered for the differential diagnosis of parkinsonian
        syndromes.   D (DS)

5.8 Magnetic resonance volumetry

Magnetic resonance volumetry uses the same principles as structural MRI to measure the size of three-dimensional volumes of tissue. This technique has been used to examine the size of various structures involved in the pathology of PD.

Can magnetic resonance volumetry be used in the differential diagnosis of parkinsonism?

5.8.1 Methodology

Two studies[76,77] addressed the diagnostic effectiveness of magnetic resonance volumetry against retrospective clinical diagnosis in determining an accurate diagnosis in people with parkinsonian syndrome.

5.8.2 Evidence statements

One study[77] (N=61) found no differences between people with PD and controls on any of the magnetic resonance volume measures. However, individuals with PSP were distinguished from people with PD and controls with a sensitivity of 95.2% and a specificity of 90.9% (mainly due to frontal grey matter volume measure). **(DS Ib)**

Another study[76] (N=53) found that mean superior cerebellar peduncle volume atrophy on visual image analysis differentiated PSP from PD, MSA and controls with a sensitivity of 74% and a specificity of 94%, whereas in quantitative analysis the best sensitivity and specificity of the volumetric analysis were 74% and 77%. **(DS II)**

5.8.3 From evidence to recommendation

While two studies suggest that volumetric MRI can help in the differentiation of PD from other types of parkinsonism, further work is required before it can be recommended.

RECOMMENDATION

R18   Magnetic resonance volumetry should not be used in the differential diagnosis of
        parkinsonian syndromes, except in the context of clinical trials.   D (DS)

5.9 Magnetic resonance spectroscopy

Proton MRS measures the concentrations of intermediary metabolites in small volumes of brain tissue. N-acetylaspartate is found in the highest concentration in neurones and their processes, whereas creatine is a marker of energy status and choline is an indicator of membrane synthesis and degradation.

Can MRS be helpful in the correct diagnosis of parkinsonism?

5.9.1 Methodology

A systematic review[78] of mixed study designs assessed the diagnostic accuracy of MRS against a clinical diagnosis of a range of parkinsonian syndromes.

5.9.2 Evidence statements

The review[78] concluded that due to the heterogeneous nature of the available evidence no comments on the variability in metabolite concentrations and ratios between people with parkinsonian disorders could safely be made. (DS II)

5.9.3 From evidence to recommendation

Contradictory results have been found on the value of MRS in differentiating PD from controls and other types of parkinsonism.

RECOMMENDATION

R19   Magnetic resonance spectroscopy should not be used in the differential diagnosis of parkinsonian syndromes.   **B (DS)**

5.10 Acute levodopa and apomorphine challenge tests

Many people with PD respond to single doses of oral levodopa and/or subcutaneous apomorphine.

Can such responses be assessed using clinical rating scales to provide a diagnostic test for PD?

5.10.1 Methodology

A systematic review[79] and an additional diagnostic study[80] addressed the effectiveness of acute levodopa and apomorphine testing in determining an accurate diagnosis of people with a parkinsonian syndrome. Another review[81] published prior to the included systematic review[79] was excluded because it summarised the same papers.

5.10.2 Evidence statements

The systematic review[79] included 13 studies, four of which examined people with de novo PD and nine others which examined people with well-established PD and with other parkinsonian syndromes. These two groups are presented separately in Table 5.7 and Table 5.8. The diagnostic study[80] followed people with PD for 3 years to investigate whether an acute challenge of carbidopa/levodopa had better diagnostic accuracy compared with the acute apomorphine challenge test. These results are also included in Table 5.8.

The systematic review used logistic regression analysis to determine whether there was a significant difference between the three tests for the misclassification of participants. Two studies[82,83] demonstrated no significant difference between the acute apomorphine challenge test and chronic levodopa therapy. However, two other studies[82,84] provided evidence that there was a difference between the acute levodopa challenge test and chronic levodopa therapy, in favour of chronic levodopa ($p<0.001$). (**DS II**)

The diagnostic study[80] commented on the adverse reactions to acute apomorphine challenges. Drowsiness, nausea, vomiting, hypotension and sweating were reported to such an extent that these effects prevented an increased dosage in some people with PD. Levodopa was better tolerated than apomorphine, with vomiting and nausea still occurring, but infrequently. No statistics were provided on whether the better tolerance of the levodopa challenge over the apomorphine challenge was significant. (**DS III**)

Table 5.7 Diagnostic accuracy of acute apomorphine and levodopa challenge testing in *de novo* PD cases[79]

Test	(N)	Positive predictive value (95% confidence interval)	Grade
Acute apomorphine (1.5–5 mg)	187	0.63 (95% CI 0.56 to 0.70)	DS II
Acute levodopa (125–275 mg)	67	0.69 (95% CI 0.59 to 0.80)	
Chronic levodopa (<1000 mg)	209	0.76 (95% CI 0.70 to 0.82)	

5.10.3 From evidence to recommendation

The evidence demonstrates that acute challenge tests with levodopa and apomorphine add nothing to standard chronic levodopa therapy in the differentiation of established cases of PD from other causes of parkinsonism. Furthermore, when used in the early stages of the disease, as they would be in clinical practice, acute challenges with levodopa and apomorphine are less discriminatory than the standard practice of treating people with levodopa as outpatients. This does not preclude the use of acute apomorphine challenges to assess whether a person with later PD will still respond to dopaminergic medication.

Table 5.8 Diagnostic accuracy of acute apomorphine and levodopa challenge testing in established PD cases[79,80]

Test	(N)		Sensitivity (%) (95% confidence interval)	Specificity (%) (95% confidence interval)	Grade
	PD	Non-PD			
Acute apomorphine 0.7–10 mg[79]	236	126	86 (95% CI 0.78 to 0.94)	85 (95% CI 0.74 to 0.96)	DS II
Acute levodopa 275 mg[79]	135	39	75 (95% CI 0.64 to 0.85)	87 (95% CI 0.77 to 0.97)	
Chronic levodopa <1000 mg[79]	155	47	91 (95% CI 0.85 to 0.99)	77 (95% CI 0.61 to 0.93)	
Acute carbidopa/ levodopa 250/25 mg[80]	83	51	77.1	71.7	DS III
Acute apomorphine	83	51			
1.5 mg[80]			70.5	65.9	
3 mg[80]			76.5	63.9	
4.5 mg[80]			76.5	66.7	

RECOMMENDATION

R20   Acute levodopa and apomorphine challenge tests should not be used in the differential diagnosis of parkinsonian syndromes.   B (DS)

5.11 Objective smell testing

Around 80% of people with PD may have an impaired sense of smell (hyposmia).[85]

Since smell can be objectively tested with a battery of different odours, is it possible that objective smell identification may be useful in PD differential diagnosis?

5.11.1 Methodology

We found six diagnostic studies looking at the effectiveness of smell testing in PD differential diagnosis. Two techniques were employed: the 'Sniffin Sticks' test[86] and the University of Pennsylvania Smell Identification Test (UPSIT). The tests were used to differentiate parkinsonian syndromes[86–88] and people with PD from healthy controls.[85,89,90]

5.11.2 Evidence statements

A separate summary of the five diagnostic accuracy studies is listed in Table 5.9 and Table 5.10. One study[90] found the discriminatory test scores decreased as a function of age for each of the participant groups and that, on average, lower UPSIT scores are needed to clinically define PD in males than in females. (**DS II**)

Another study[89] reported that of the 40 odorants in the UPSIT test, the combined smell of pizza and wintergreen was the best discriminator. In addition, pizza (oregano smell) alone specifically indicates anosmia for people with PD with a very high sensitivity and specificity (Table 5.10). (**DS II**)

A third study[85] found abnormal olfactory function in 82% of the PD participants tested compared with 23% of controls. (**DS II**)

Table 5.9 Diagnostic accuracy of smell-testing techniques in differentiating parkinsonian syndromes							
Technique	**Groups (N)**	**Mean age (years)**	**Disease duration (years)**	**Cut-off score**	**Sensitivity (%)**	**Specificity (%)**	**Grade**
'Sniffin Sticks'[86]	PD (7) versus MSA (8)	57.7	5.8	19.5 24.8	78 100	100 63	DS Ib
UPSIT test[87]	PD (118) versus MSA (29), PSP (15) and CBD (7)	59.4 63.7	–	25	77	85	DS III
UPSIT test[91]	PD (18) versus VP (14)	70.6 74.1	9.1 6.6	>22	85.7	88.9	DS II
UPSIT test[91]	PD (NR) versus VP (8)	65–75	–	≤23	100	85.7	DS II
UPSIT test[91]	PD (NR) versus VP (6)	76–88	–	≤22	85.7	80	DS II

VP = vascular parkinsonism; NR = not reported.

Table 5.10 Diagnostic accuracy of smell-testing techniques in differentiating parkinsonian syndromes from non-parkinsonian syndromes

Technique	Groups (N)	Mean age (years)	Disease duration (years)	Cut-off score	Sensitivity (%)	Specificity (%)	Grade
B-SIT test[85]	PD (49) versus control (52)	68 71	5	–	82	82	DS II
UPSIT test[90]	Male: PD (52) versus controls (76)	61 to 70	5 (3 months-48 years)	25	81	82	DS II
UPSIT test[90]	Female: PD (20) versus control (104)	61 to 70	See above	30	80	88	DS II
UPSIT test[90]	Male: PD (32) versus controls (128)	≤60	See above	31	91	88	DS II
UPSIT test[90]	Female: PD (28) versus control (112)	≤60	See above	33	79	85	DS II
UPSIT test[90]	Male: PD (25) versus controls (100)	≥71	See above	22	76	78	DS II
UPSIT test[90]	Female: PD (23) versus control (92)	≥71	See above	25	78	82	DS II
Pizza and wintergreen[89]	IPD (96) versus controls (96)	62	Not stated	NA	90	86	DS II
Pizza (oregano smell) only[89]		45.6			76	90	DS II

5.11.3 From evidence to recommendation

Objective smell testing has a moderate sensitivity and specificity in differentiating people with PD from controls. However, there are few data on its ability to differentiate PD from other parkinsonian syndromes. Smell is also diminished in Alzheimer's disease.[92] At present, smell identification adds little in the differential diagnosis of parkinsonism but this situation may change with further research.

RECOMMENDATION

R21   Objective smell testing should not be used in the differential diagnosis of parkinsonian syndromes, except in the context of clinical trials.   B (DS)

6 | Neuroprotection

6.1 | Definitions

Neuroprotection is a process in which a treatment beneficially affects the underlying pathophysiology of PD (Figure 6.1). This definition is preferred to 'disease-modifying therapy' since the latter may encompass processes, which lead to modification of clinical outcomes without any effect on the underlying pathophysiology of the condition. Good examples of this are drugs that delay the onset of motor complications in PD, such as dopamine agonists. This outcome is not necessarily due to a neuroprotective effect; it may arise from a variety of pharmacokinetic and pharmacodynamic mechanisms.[93,94]

Neurorescue refers to the salvage of dying neurones; this may mean a stabilising of the condition with prevention of further cell loss rather than any progressive increase in cell number (Figure 6.1).[93,94]

Neurorestoration refers to increasing the numbers of dopaminergic neurones by techniques such as cell implantation and nerve growth factor infusion (Figure 6.1). Such surgical techniques are discussed but not reviewed in the chapter on 'Surgery for Parkinson's disease'.[93,94]

Neuromodulation has been used by some to refer to deep brain stimulation (DBS) procedures in PD such as bilateral subthalamic stimulation.[93,94]

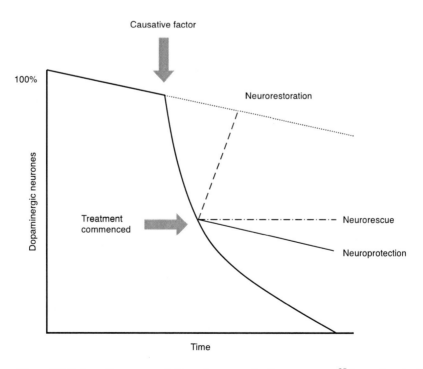

Figure 6.1 Schematic representation of neuroprotective processes[95] (reproduced with permission from the authors)

6.1.1 Pathogenesis of disease modification

Detailed discussion of this topic is beyond the scope of this guideline.[96] However, the main pathophysiological mechanisms upon which agents may be neuroprotective are listed below:

- mitochondrial complex-1 deficiency
- free radical damage and oxidative stress
- proteasomal dysfunction
- apoptosis
- inflammation (microglial activation).

6.1.2 Measuring disease progression

Considerable debate surrounds how to measure the rate of progression of PD in clinical trials of neuroprotective therapies.[93,97] The measures used to date are detailed in Table 6.1 along with a summary of their potential benefits and drawbacks.

Table 6.1 Outcome measures used in neuroprotection trials in PD		
Outcome measures	**Benefits**	**Problems**
Quality of life	Patient-rated so more meaningful to them.	Open to symptomatic effects of therapy. Likely to have low sensitivity unless agent has large treatment effect.
Clinical rating scales	Standard method used for many years.	Open to symptomatic effects of therapy unless evaluated after drug withdrawal.
Mortality	Has direct relevance to people with PD.	Open to symptomatic effects of therapy. Studies need to be large or long term to have adequate power.
SPECT and PET imaging	Intuitively a good biomarker for the disease. May improve diagnostic accuracy at start of trials. May be more sensitive than clinical outcomes.	People who have PD clinically but have normal baseline scan. People with PD with abnormal baseline radionuclide studies may have PSP or MSA. Lack of clinical correlation of neuroprotection in radionuclide studies to date. Poor sensitivity to change and reproducibility of radionuclide studies. Differential regulation of ligand pharmacokinetics by medication.
Delaying motor complications	Has direct relevance to people with PD.	More likely to be a pharmacokinetic or dynamic effect than neuroprotection.

Adapted from Refs 97,98.

The majority of previous neuroprotection trials have been of parallel group design and placebo controlled. A washout period at the end of the study was often included to remove the symptomatic effects of the active agent. In general, clinical rating scales have been seen as the most acceptable measure of disease modification. One study used a delayed-start design to reduce the numbers of people with PD given placebo.[99] With this technique one group is randomised to active treatment from the outset but one or more other groups are randomised to start the active drug after a period on placebo (Figure 6.2). If the drug has a symptomatic effect then clinical outcome measures in the groups will merge together, given sufficient follow-up. If the drug delays disease progression then clinical ratings will remain different between the groups.

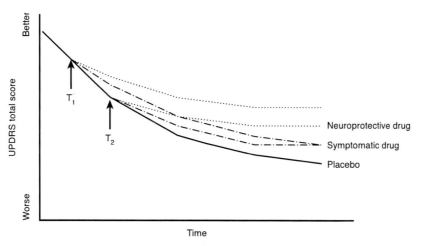

Figure 6.2 Schematic representation of delayed-start design trial.[94]

At time points T_1 and T_2 people with PD are randomised to drug or placebo.

With neuroprotective drugs, outcome scores will be parallel but with drugs that have a symptomatic effect the curves come together.[94]

6.1.3 Methodological limitations of neuroprotective studies

When reviewing the evidence on neuroprotective agents, the following methodological issues should be considered:

- wide range in sample size
- lack of statistical detail on power of small studies
- no documentation of allocation concealment methods
- comparability of results from different centres in multi-site studies
- drug regimen varied between trials (drug, dose, frequency).

6.1.4 Potential neuroprotective agents

Many agents suggested to have neuroprotective properties have undergone systematic review by the National Institute for Neurologic Disorders and Stroke (NINDS).[100] They developed a shortlist of 12 candidate drugs for neuroprotection trials, which are listed in Table 6.2. In addition, vitamin E has been examined for neuroprotective potential.

On the basis of the evidence available, the GDG chose to review the four classes of potential neuroprotective drugs for PD based on the human studies:

- vitamins
- co-enzyme Q_{10}
- dopamine agonists
- monoamine oxidase type B (MAOB) inhibitors.

Table 6.2 Candidate neuroprotective drugs for PD selected by NINDS[100]	
Caffeine	Minocycline
Co-enzyme Q_{10}	Nicotine
Creatine	Oestrogen
GM-1 ganglioside	Monoamine oxidase type B inhibitors (rasagiline and selegiline)
GPi-1485	Dopamine agonists (ropinirole and pramipexole)

6.2 Vitamin E

If the generation of free radicals is a significant pathophysiological process in PD, then the anti-oxidant vitamins E and C may be neuroprotective. No trials with vitamin C have been done in PD.

Does vitamin E have neuroprotective properties in PD?

6.2.1 Methodology

Three papers[101–103] were found, which analysed data from the same cohort recruited into the DATATOP study.[104] The DATATOP study (N=800) was a randomised controlled study, which addressed whether vitamin E (tocopherol 2000 IU) was effective in reducing the progression of PD.

6.2.2 Evidence statements

All of the studies[101–103] failed to demonstrate a significant benefit of vitamin E in slowing the progression of PD. (1++)

One report[101] examined 24 months' follow-up data and showed the following:
- The probability of reaching the endpoint (onset of disability prompting administration of levodopa) was not reduced in people with PD receiving tocopherol.
- There was no significant change in UPDRS variables for the tocopherol treatment groups.
- There was no evidence of any beneficial effect of α-tocopherol (2000 IU per day) in either slowing functional decline or ameliorating the clinical features of PD. (1++)

Another report[103] looked at 24 months' follow-up data and showed:
- no significant benefit of tocopherol in reducing the likelihood of reaching the endpoint (requiring levodopa therapy)
- no significant benefit on any of the secondary outcome measures (UPDRS, Hoehn and Yahr scale, Schwab and England Activities of Daily Living (ADL) scale, neuropsychological testing, Hamilton depression scale). (1++)

A third report[102] looked at 14 months' follow-up data and showed no significant effects for tocopherol on the annualised rates of change of any cognitive measure after adjustment for multiple comparisons. (1+)

6.2.3 From evidence to recommendation

The DATATOP evidence shows that vitamin E taken as 2000 IU of tocopherol daily is not neuroprotective in PD.

RECOMMENDATION

R22   Vitamin E should not be used as a neuroprotective therapy for people with PD.   **A**

6.3 Co-enzyme Q$_{10}$

Mitochondrial complex I activity is reduced in post-mortem substantia nigra and in the platelets of people with PD.[105,106] Co-enzyme Q$_{10}$ is the electron acceptor for complexes I and II and as a result is a potent anti-oxidant. The level of co-enzyme Q$_{10}$ is reduced in platelet mitochondria in PD.[107] Oral supplementation with co-enzyme Q$_{10}$ reduced dopaminergic neurone loss in MPTP-treated mice.[108]

In view of this positive pre-clinical work, is there any clinical trial evidence that co-enzyme Q$_{10}$ has neuroprotective properties in PD?

6.3.1 Methodology

Two studies[109,110] examined the effectiveness of co-enzyme Q$_{10}$ in reducing the rate of progression of PD. The methodological limitations included a lack of detail concerning randomisation and allocation concealment in one study,[109] and a small sample size without power calculations in both studies.[109,110]

6.3.2 Evidence statements

The two studies[109,110] used validated clinical rating scales as the outcome measures to assess benefit from co-enzyme Q$_{10}$.

One trial[110] (N=80) compared three different doses (300 mg/d, 600 mg/d and 1,200 mg/d) of co-enzyme Q$_{10}$ with placebo using total UPDRS scale as the primary outcome measure. The primary analysis was a test for trend between placebo and all doses of co-enzyme Q$_{10}$. This showed a significant difference (5.30; 95% CI 0.21 to 10.39) at the p=0.09 level. In a pre-specified secondary analysis, which compared each of the dosages to placebo, only the 1,200 mg/d group had a significant effect compared with placebo (p=0.04). (1++)

This trial[110] also found the following.

* People with PD taking co-enzyme Q$_{10}$ displayed a worsening on the Schwab and England scale as assessed by the examiner (p=0.04) but not by the person with PD (p=0.81).
* Co-enzyme Q$_{10}$ did not have a significant effect on the scores for the Hoehn and Yahr scale or the timed tapping task. (1++)

Another trial[109] (N=28) compared a low dose (360 mg/day) of co-enzyme Q_{10} with placebo and showed:

- the UPDRS total score was in favour of co-enzyme Q_{10} treatment (p=0.012)
- a benefit of co-enzyme Q_{10} supplementation on the Visual Function Test (p=0.008) measured with the Farnsworth–Munsell 100 Hue Test. (1+)

6.3.3 From evidence to recommendation

The small neuroprotection trials performed with co-enzyme Q_{10} in PD so far have been encouraging, but further evidence is required before it can be recommended routinely.

RECOMMENDATION

R23   Co-enzyme Q_{10} should not be used as a neuroprotective therapy for people with PD, except in the context of clinical trials.   **B**

6.4 Dopamine agonists

A considerable body of pre-clinical work has suggested that dopamine agonists are neuro-protective in cell culture and various animal models of PD.[111,112]

What clinical evidence is there that dopamine agonists have neuroprotective properties in PD?

6.4.1 Methodology

Eight studies[42,61,113–118] were found which addressed the neuroprotective effects of dopamine agonists versus levodopa therapy in PD.

One trial[114] was excluded due to the lack of reporting drug dosages used during the trial, which limits the comparability with other trials to show consistency of effect.

GDG members found a related abstract[119] on pergolide therapy, but this abstract was excluded, as the results have not been published in a full paper.

Of the six studies included in the evidence base, half of them were designed as open trials. Usually, this would be a serious methodological issue as open trials are subject to increased performance bias. However, one of the main outcome measures was mortality, which cannot be influenced by the open-trial design. In addition, the long-term follow-up of 4.5 and 10 years is practical justification for an open-trial design.[42,117,115]

There were specific methodological issues associated with the imaging studies. One study reported at baseline that 11% of the people who had been clinically diagnosed with PD had normal scans.[61] Another study did not include a washout period in order to distinguish between the symptomatic and neuroprotective effects of the drugs administered.[113]

6.4.2   Evidence statements

With respect to clinical rating scales, the ropinirole REAL-PET (N=162) study found UPDRS motor score during treatment at 2 years was superior with levodopa compared with ropinirole (a score increase of 0.70 in the ropinirole group and a decrease of 5.64 in the levodopa group, 95% CI 3.54 to 9.14).[61] (1++)

Non-significant results reported by the studies included:

* CALM-PD[113] (pramipexole) (N=82) mean total and mean motor UPDRS (1++)
* REAL-PET[61] (ropinirole) Clinical Global Impression (CGI) improvement scale (1++)
* UK-PDRG study[42] (bromocriptine) (N=782) mean Webster disability scores (1+)
* cabergoline study[118] UPDRS part III (motor) (N=412) and part II (ADL). (1+)

With respect to mortality, the following results were found.

* The PRADO study[115] (N=587) was terminated when 18 deaths were reported in the levodopa group versus eight deaths in the levodopa/bromocriptine group (p=0.07; adjusted for age and sex p=0.02). The risk ratio of death in the levodopa group compared with the levodopa/bromocriptine group was 2.7, a reduction of 63%. (1+)
* All three of the bromocriptine studies[53,116,117] found no significant differences between treatment groups. (1+)
* The cabergoline study[118] found no significant difference between treatment groups. (1+)

With respect to imaging, several analytical measures found benefit of ropinirole and pramipexole over levodopa; these are summarised in Table 6.3.

Table 6.3 Rate of decline in tracer uptake (1++)

Variable	% Change dopamine agonist	% Change levodopa	Significance
Ropinirole (REAL-PET)[61]	(SE)	(SE)	
Region-of-interest analysis (reduction in putamen Ki over 2 years)	13.4% (2.14)	20.3% (2.35)	RD 34% (95% CI 0.65 to 13.06, p=0.022)
Statistical parametric mapping (reduction in putamen)	14.1% (1.58)	22.9% (1.70)	RD 38% (95% CI 4.24 to 13.3, p<0.005)
Amplitudes of change (substantia nigra)	4.3 % (3.67)	−7.5 % (3.94)	MD 11.9 (95% CI 1.3 to 22.4, p=0.025)
Pramipexole (CALM-PD)[113]	(SD)	(SD)	
Striatal ^{123}I-β-CIT (rate of decline) at 22 months	−7.1 (9.0)	−13.5 (9.6)	p=0.004
At 34 months	−10.9 (11.8)	−19.6 (12.4)	p=0.009
At 46 months	−16.0 (13.3)	−25.5 (14.1)	p=0.01

RD = relative difference; Ki = influx constant; SE= standard error; MD= mean difference.

With respect to motor complications:

- the REAL-PET study[61] found:
  - development of dyskinesia favoured ropinirole (odds ratio (OR) 0.09, 95% CI 0.02 to 0.29, p<0.001)
  - time to develop dyskinesias favoured ropinirole (hazard ratio 8.28, 95% CI 2.46 to 27.93, p<0.001) (1++)
- the PRADO study[115] found the incidence of dyskinesias favoured bromocriptine (rate ratio: 0.73, 95% CI 0.57 to 0.93). (1+)

The cabergoline versus levodopa study[118] found:

- risk of developing motor complications favoured cabergoline treatment (p<0.02)
- the relative risk of developing motor complications was >50% lower with cabergoline compared with levodopa
- cabergoline-treated people requiring levodopa were at the same risk of developing motor complications as those on a stable levodopa dose. (1+)

6.4.3 From evidence to recommendation

The apparent reduction in the rate of tracer loss in the ropinirole and pramipexole trials shown by radionuclide imaging raised the prospect that these agonists are neuroprotective. However, there are a number of methodological problems with these studies (as shown in Table 6.1).[97] Clinical motor rating scales were better in levodopa-treated individuals with PD or no different in these trials. The delaying of motor complications by the agonists may be due to a pharmacokinetic or pharmacodynamic effect rather than slowing of disease progression.

RECOMMENDATION

R24   Dopamine agonists should not be used as neuroprotective therapies for people with PD, except in the context of clinical trials.   B

6.5   Monoamine oxidase type B inhibitors

The propargylamines selegiline and rasagiline are monoamine oxidase type B (MAOB) inhibitors, thereby reducing the turnover of dopamine and hopefully reducing free radical generation.[96] However, they may also have an anti-apoptotic effect.[100]

What *in vivo* evidence is there that MAOB inhibitors are neuroprotective in PD?

6.5.1 Methodology

Two meta-analyses[120,121] and an RCT[99] were found, which addressed the effectiveness of MAOB inhibitors in reducing the rate of progression of PD.

One meta-analysis included 3,525 people with PD in 17 randomised trials; 13 trials were on selegiline, three trials were on lazabemide and one trial was on rasagiline therapy. Only selegiline and rasagiline are licensed for use in the UK. The results of the lazabemide studies were consistent with the results of the other two therapies, so the full meta-analysis was included in the evidence base. The other meta-analysis[121] was a Cochrane review with a similar authorship. This included 2,422 people with PD from 10 trials where treatment duration or follow-up was 1 year or longer. Nine trials were on selegiline and one was on lazabemide. Several trials were included in both meta-analyses.

The RCT[99] consisted of 404 people with PD randomised to rasagiline or placebo-delayed rasagiline therapy. The delayed-start design (see Figure 6.2) consisted of randomising them to one of three groups:

- rasagiline 1 mg/d for 1 year
- rasagiline 2 mg/d for 1 year
- placebo for 6 months, followed by rasagiline 2 mg/d for 6 months.

6.5.2 Evidence statements

A meta-analysis[120] combined the available data from six trials of selegiline therapy. All trials showed significantly improved scores in favour of selegiline versus controls for UPDRS scores at 3 months as follows:

- total score: 2.7 (95% CI 1.4 to 4.1, p=0.00009)
- motor score: 1.8 (95% CI 0.8 to 2.7, p=0.0004)
- activities of daily living scores: 0.9 points (95% CI 0.5 to 1.4, p=0.00007).

The Cochrane review[121] also found significantly improved scores in favour of MAOB inhibitors from baseline to 1 year on treatment. (1++)

Although the large DATATOP study accounted for over 79% of people with PD in a MAOB inhibitors versus placebo comparison, the combined results from the other studies were consistent with those from DATATOP (p=0.004).[120] (1++)

The rasagiline trial[99] showed:

- Total UPDRS score for rasagiline 1 mg/d for 1 year versus delayed-start rasagiline 2 mg/d for 6 months was significant −1.82 (95% CI 3.64 to 0.001, p=0.05) in favour of longer treatment.
- Rasagiline 2 mg/d for 1 year versus delayed-start rasagiline 2 mg/d for 6 months was significant −2.29 (95% CI −4.11 to −0.48, p=0.01) in favour of longer treatment.
- ADL score for rasagiline 2 mg/d for 1 year versus delayed-start rasagiline 2 mg/d for 6 months significantly favoured the longer treatment (p=0.005).
- The comparisons of other UPDRS subscales were not significant. (1++)

A meta-analysis[120] assessed mortality rates by combining all of the available data from nine trials of selegiline and one trial of lazabemide therapy. The results in eight trials (excluding UK-PDRG), showed:

- no excess in mortality between MAOB inhibitor-treated individuals with PD and controls (p=0.8)
- in the UK-PDRG study there were significantly more deaths in the selegiline arm versus the levodopa arm (OR=1.57, 95% CI 1.09 to 2.30, p=0.015)
- by taking all available data, 20% of deaths occurred in the MAOB inhibitor group compared with 21% in the controls (p=0.2)

- no significant heterogeneity was found between trials (p=0.6), even including the UK-PDRG study
- the Cochrane review[121] found a non-significant increase in deaths among patients treated with MAOB inhibitors compared with controls. (1++)

A meta-analysis[120] found five trials, which reported data on motor complications. The combined results showed:

- a 25% reduction in motor fluctuations in MAOB inhibitor group (0.75, 95% CI 0.59 to 0.95, p=0.02).
- no difference in the incidence of dyskinesia between treatment groups (0.97, 95% CI 0.75 to 1.26, p=0.8) compared with non-MAOB inhibitor group.

The Cochrane review[121] found very similar results. However, with regard to motor fluctuations, they found that the result was dependent on the adjusted results of one study (the UK-PDRG study) and if the unadjusted figures were used the overall result became insignificant. Additionally, results were not reported for a number of patients in these studies and a modified worst-case sensitivity analysis also made the results non-significant. (1++)

6.5.3 From evidence to recommendation

The benefits of MAOB inhibitors versus control in terms of clinical rating scales were consistent with a known short-term symptomatic effect. There does not seem to be any clear increase or decrease in mortality with MAOB inhibitors. The delayed onset of motor fluctuations with MAOB inhibitors is comparable to the delayed motor complications with dopamine agonists but is likely to represent a levodopa-sparing effect involving pharmacokinetic or pharmacodynamic factors.

The sustained difference in total UPDRS in the rasagiline versus placebo delayed-start design trial suggests this agent may be neuroprotective. However, the relatively short follow-up in this trial may not have been long enough to see the UPDRS scores in the different trial groups merge, as would be seen with a symptomatic effect.

Further large trials with longer-term follow-up are required to assess whether the MAOB inhibitors have neuroprotective properties in PD.

RECOMMENDATION

R25   MAOB inhibitors should not be used as neuroprotective therapies for people with PD, except in the context of clinical trials.   B

7 | Symptomatic pharmacological therapy in Parkinson's disease

7.1 Introduction

Symptomatic therapies for PD treat the symptoms of the disease but do not necessarily slow the rate of progression of the condition. In this guideline the symptomatic pharmacological therapies have been classified on the basis of the clinical manifestations of a person with PD. Thus:

- Early disease has been used to refer to people with PD who have developed functional disability and require symptomatic therapy.
- Later disease has been used to refer to people on levodopa who have developed motor complications.

Clinical trials and regulatory authorities define the term 'later disease' in the same way. However, since motor complications can occur soon after starting levodopa, particularly if large doses are used, 'later disease' is something of a misnomer. The term is generally preferred to the alternative 'advanced disease'.

7.1.1 Methodological limitations of symptomatic therapy studies

When reviewing the symptomatic therapy evidence, the following methodological issues should be considered:

- trial duration is often too short
- drug regimen variations between trials (type of drug, dose, frequency)
- small sample size which limits generalisability and sensitivity of tests to detect outcome differences between groups
- lack of reporting methods of randomisation and allocation concealment
- lack of washout periods between treatment arms in crossover studies
- lack of reporting results of first arm from crossover studies, which leads to risk of carry-over effect
- lack of intention-to-treat analyses
- lack of defining the clinical criteria for diagnosis
- clinical versus statistical significance
- over-representation of younger patients limiting generalisability.

Most of the poorly designed trials were performed in the 1970s and 1980s when trial design was in its infancy. Drugs evaluated in such trials may not have been found to be efficacious in this review. However, this does not mean that they are ineffective. In such cases, clinical experience may be the only appropriate judge of efficacy and safety.

The Cochrane reviews included in this chapter have received a 1++ grading for the methodology of the systematic review as applied by the Cochrane group, but this grading does not apply to the trials contained within these reviews. Although the methodologies of the systematic reviews were of good quality, the trials contained within the reviews sometimes suffered from methodological limitations. The results of these trials should be treated with caution due to the inherent methodological limitations. In light of this, it was felt to be inappropriate to present evidence statements based on the individual trial data.

Efficacy outcome measures in later disease trials are considerably different from those in early disease. The people with PD in such trials have already developed motor complications and the aim of adjuvant therapy is to reduce the time the person with PD spends 'off' and to reduce the dose of levodopa, which has played some part in the generation of the complications in the first place. 'Off' time is measured from patient-completed 30 minute epoch 'on'/'off' diary cards, which are usually averaged over a 3-day period. Levodopa dose is recorded throughout the trial. Usually the UPDRS scale components are also noted during later disease trials.

7.2 Early pharmacological therapy

7.2.1 Introduction

It was evident from reviewing the evidence-base that there is no single drug of choice in the initial pharmacotherapy of early PD. Table 7.1 may help to guide the reader through the following section.

Table 7.1 Options for initial pharmacotherapy in early PD				
	First-choice option	Symptom control	Possible risk of side effects	
			Motor complications	Other adverse events
Levodopa	✓	+++	↑	↑
Dopamine agonists	✓	++	↓	↑
MAOB inhibitors	✓	+	↓	↑
Anticholinergics	✗	Lack of evidence	Lack of evidence	Lack of evidence
Beta-blockers	✗	Lack of evidence	Lack of evidence	Lack of evidence
Amantadine	✗	Lack of evidence	Lack of evidence	Lack of evidence

+++ = Good degree of symptom control.
++ = Moderate degree of symptom control.
+ = Limited degree of symptom control.
↑ = Evidence of increased motor complications/other adverse events.
↓ = Evidence of reduced motor complications/other adverse events.

7.2.2 Levodopa

The standard symptomatic therapy for PD for more than 30 years has been levodopa. This is the precursor of dopamine which is deficient in PD. Levodopa is readily converted into dopamine by dopa decarboxylase. To reduce peripheral metabolism of levodopa, it is combined with a peripheral dopa decarboxylase inhibitor (ie carbidopa or benserazide). This increases the amount of levodopa that crosses the blood-brain barrier.

However, levodopa preparations contribute to the development of motor complications in PD. These comprise abnormal involuntary movements or dyskinesias, such as athetosis and dystonia, along with response fluctuations in which people experience 'wearing off' of the drug's effects and/or unpredictable switching between the 'on' and the 'off' state.

To avoid motor complications, the strategy of delaying the introduction of levodopa has developed. Most people with PD who commence therapy with another drug will eventually need levodopa therapy. This approach requires initial therapy with an alternative that is as effective as levodopa that does not cause motor complications. A number of drug classes have been examined for such properties.

▷ Methodology

Only one RCT[62] (ELLDOPA) was found which addressed the effectiveness of levodopa (plus a decarboxylase inhibitor) compared with placebo. The other trials found included studies on levodopa monotherapy compared with placebo and were published between 1969 and 1971. These were not reviewed, as levodopa is no longer used without a decarboxylase inhibitor.

The RCT[62] was a large multi-centre study including 361 early PD people randomly assigned to four groups, consisting of three different doses of levodopa/carbidopa (150/37.5 mg/day, 300/75 mg/day or 600/150 mg/day) or placebo.

All people included in the trial had received a diagnosis of PD within the last 2 years and no one was on any anti-parkinsonian medication at the time of enrolment. The trial duration was 40 weeks, which was followed by a 2-week withdrawal period at the end of the trial.

There were two primary outcome measures: clinical assessment using UPDRS and measurement of the dopamine transporter with ^{123}I-β-CIT SPECT.

▷ Evidence statements

With respect to clinical rating scales:[62]
* Levodopa in a dose-dependent pattern reduced the worsening of symptoms of PD.
* Changes in UPDRS scores from baseline to week 42 (versus placebo) were:
    – total score ($p < 0.001$)
    – ADL component ($p < 0.001$)
    – motor component ($p < 0.01$)
    – mental component (non-significant).
* The UPDRS scores in the three levodopa groups worsened during the 2-week washout period but did not deteriorate to placebo levels.
* The group receiving the highest dose of levodopa had the largest improvement in UPDRS. (1++)

With respect to ^{123}I-β-CIT (neuroimaging) outcomes:[62]
* The percentage decrease in striatal ^{123}I-β-CIT uptake over 40 weeks was greater among participants in the levodopa than the placebo group and, although this was non-significant, 15% of people had a putaminal uptake of more than 75% of that of age-matched controls.

- Analysis of the results after exclusion of the 19 people without dopaminergic deficit on imaging showed a significantly greater decrease in uptake among those receiving levodopa than those receiving placebo (p=0.036). (1++)

With respect to adverse events:[62]

- Side effects were more common in the 600 mg group than with placebo for dyskinesias (p<0.001), nausea (p=0.001), infection (p=0.01), hypertonia (p=0.03), and headache (p=0.03).
- Other findings were non-significant between other levodopa doses and placebo. (1++)

With respect to withdrawal rates:[62]

- Of the total of 361 participants enrolled, 317 (88%) took the study medication for 40 weeks and 311 (86%) completed the 2 weeks of washout.
- The percentage of dropouts per group included: placebo (22%), 150 mg/d (15%), 300 mg/d (6%) and 600 mg/d (11%).
- The main reasons for withdrawal were worsening of symptoms and adverse events. (1++)

▷ From evidence to recommendations

The clinical impression that levodopa is a most effective treatment for PD has been confirmed in the large ELLDOPA trial. Short-term dopaminergic adverse effects are infrequent and usually settle with time. However, long-term levodopa therapy precipitates motor complications such as dyskinesias and motor fluctuations. Questions remain regarding the possibility that levodopa may be toxic or even protective to the remaining nigrostriatal dopaminergic neurones. Further work is required to clarify this issue.

RECOMMENDATIONS

R26   Levodopa may be used as a symptomatic treatment for people with early PD.   A

R27   The dose of levodopa should be kept as low as possible to maintain good function in order to reduce the development of motor complications.   A

7.2.3   Dopamine agonists

The dopamine receptor agonists mimic the effect of dopamine by binding directly with the post-synaptic dopamine receptors. They were introduced as adjuvant therapy to levodopa in later disease, but, more recently, trials have examined their effects as initial monotherapy in the hope that they may delay the onset of motor complications.

What is the effectiveness of dopamine agonists compared with placebo in the treatment of functionally disabled early PD?

▷ Methodology

Six randomised controlled trials[122–127] were found which compared the effectiveness of dopamine agonists with placebo for the treatment of people with early PD who are functionally disabled. The sample size for most of these studies was quite large (range N=55–335, mean 177).

▷ Evidence statements

The following outcomes were reported to be significantly in favour of dopamine agonists:

- UPDRS total score[122,123]
- UPDRS motor scores[122,124–127]
- UPDRS > 30% reduction in motor scores[122,124,127]
- UPDRS ADL scores[122,125,126]
- Schwab and England ADL scores[122]
- CGI 'very much improved' score[122,124,127]
- requirement of levodopa supplementation[124]
- withdrawal rates.[124] (1+)

The following adverse events were found to be significantly increased (p<0.05) in the treatment group:

- nausea[122,125,127]
- somnolence[122,125,127]
- dizziness[122,127]
- insomnia, constipation, hallucinations[125]
- anorexia, vomiting.[122] (1+)

The following outcomes were reported as non-significant:

- incidence of reporting adverse events[122–127]
- incidence of withdrawals.[122,127] (1+)

▷ From evidence to recommendation

Dopamine agonists are an effective treatment for the motor features of early PD. However, agonists generate significant dopaminergic adverse events. The latter do not lead to drug withdrawal, which suggests that they are mild and that tolerance develops. These conclusions apply to the relatively young people included in these studies. Further work on the efficacy and safety of dopamine agonists in older people is required.

Ergot-derived dopamine agonists (bromocriptine, cabergoline, lisuride and pergolide) are well known to cause rare serosal reactions such as pleural, pericardial and peritoneal effusion and/or fibrosis.[128] Recently, two echocardiographic series have suggested that pergolide can also cause a cardiac valvulopathy.[129,130] As a result of these reports, the pergolide Summary of Product Characteristics has been changed to include the following.

- Pergolide is to be used as second line after a non-ergot dopamine agonist.
- The dose of pergolide should not exceed 5 mg per day.
- An echocardiogram must be obtained before initiating therapy and should be repeated regularly thereafter to monitor for valvulopathy.
- Pergolide is contraindicated in anyone with anatomical evidence of cardiac valvulopathy.

Reports of serosal reactions with non-ergot dopamine agonists (pramipexole and ropinirole) are few and these are possibly due to previous exposure to ergot-derived agonists. However, the patient-years of exposure to these newer agonists is low, so firm conclusions cannot be reached.

RECOMMENDATIONS

R28   Dopamine agonists may be used as a symptomatic treatment for people with early PD.   **A**

R29   A dopamine agonist should be titrated to a clinically efficacious dose. If side effects prevent this, another agonist or a drug from another class should be used in its place.   **D (GPP)**

R30   If an ergot-derived dopamine agonist is used, the patient should have a minimum of renal function tests, erythrocyte sedimentation rate (ESR) and chest radiograph performed before starting treatment, and annually thereafter.*   **D (GPP)**

R31   In view of the monitoring required with ergot-derived dopamine agonists, a non-ergot-derived agonist should be preferred in most cases.   **D (GPP)**

7.2.4   Monoamine oxidase type B inhibitors

MAOB inhibitors block the metabolism of dopamine, thereby increasing its level in the striatum. MAOB inhibitors do not cause a reaction after consumption of tyramine-rich foods ('tyramine' or 'cheese' effect) and are therefore safer to use than non-selective inhibitors.

MAOB inhibitors were introduced as a symptomatic therapy in later PD. After encouraging pre-clinical and one retrospective clinical trial[131] they were used for a time in early PD in the hope that they might have a neuroprotective effect in addition to a symptomatic effect (see Chapter 6).

What is the evidence that MAOB inhibitors are an effective and safe symptomatic treatment in early PD?

▷   Methodology

Two meta-analyses[120,121] and two RCTs[132,133] which addressed the effectiveness of MAOB inhibitors in treating people with early PD were included.

One meta-analysis[120] included 3,525 people with PD from 17 randomised trials; 13 trials were on selegiline, three trials were on lazabemide and one trial was on rasagiline therapy. Although only selegiline and rasagiline are licensed for use in the UK, the results of the lazabemide studies were consistent with the results of the other two therapies. Thus, the meta-analysis, which combined the results of all MAOB inhibitor trials, was included in the evidence base. All of the selegiline trials used the standard oral preparation rather than the lyophilised buccal preparation selegiline (Zelapar®). The other meta-analysis[121] was a Cochrane review with a similar authorship. This included 2,422 people with PD from 10 trials where treatment duration or follow-up was 1 year or longer. Nine trials were on selegiline and one was on lazabemide. Several trials were included in both meta-analyses.

One RCT[133] consisted of 15 people with PD. The small sample size could explain the non-significant results, when compared with the large meta-analysis. The other RCT[132] consisted of 56 people with PD, divided into three rasagiline dose groups (1, 2 or 4 mg/d) and a placebo group. The authors of this study reported that the trial was inadequately powered for assessing anti-parkinsonian efficacy of the study drug.

---

*Full details of the restrictions on pergolide use and monitoring are available in the Summary of Product Characteristics.

▷ Evidence statements

The large DATATOP study accounted for over 65% of the people with PD analysed for UPDRS scores and over 79% of people with PD in the MAOB inhibitor versus placebo comparison. The combined results from the other two studies of MAOB inhibitor compared with placebo were consistent with those from DATATOP and were significant independently (p=0.004).[120] (1++)

With respect to clinical rating scales, one meta-analysis[120] reported:
- UPDRS scores at 3 months from six trials (all used selegiline for MAOB inhibitor intervention) were:
  - total score: treatment difference 2.7 (95% CI 1.4 to 4.1, p=0.00009)
  - motor score: treatment difference 1.8 (95% CI 0.8 to 2.7, p=0.0004)
  - ADL score: treatment difference 0.9 (95% CI 0.5 to 1.4, p=0.00007).
- All of the above quoted outcomes favoured selegiline over controls.

The Cochrane review[121] also found that MAOB inhibitors significantly improved these UPDRS scores. (1++)

The randomised crossover trial[133] reported no significant differences on the Webster rating scale (total scores) for people with PD on co-beneldopa/selegiline compared with people with PD on co-beneldopa/placebo. (1++)

The other RCT[132] reported:
- Total UPDRS score during 10-week period (p<0.05) for rasagiline 2 mg but not for 1 mg and 4 mg groups compared with placebo.
- A responder analysis showed that 28% of people (12/43) receiving rasagiline had an improvement in total UPDRS score of more than 30%, compared with none of the people receiving placebo (p<0.05).
- No evidence of drug effect was noted with respect to the Clinician's Global Impression of Change (CGIC) scale, Hoehn and Yahr stage, Schwab and England ADL scale, or BDI. (1++)

With respect to need for levodopa therapy, the meta-analysis[120] found the following:
- Eight trials reported data on the need for levodopa (MAOB inhibitor versus placebo). The combination of these trial results showed a highly significant reduction in need for levodopa in people with PD randomised to a MAOB inhibitor compared with placebo (0.57, 95% CI 0.48 to 0.67, p<0.00001).

The Cochrane review[121] found a similar significant reduction in the requirement for levodopa, although it was noted that all patients were receiving levodopa after 4 years of follow-up. (1++)

With respect to motor complications, one meta-analysis[120] found five trials. The combined results showed:
- 25% reduction in motor fluctuations in MAOB inhibitor group, treatment difference 0.75 (95% CI 0.59 to 0.95, p=0.02)
- no significant difference in the incidence of dyskinesia between treatment groups compared with non-MAOB inhibitor group.

The Cochrane review[121] found very similar results. However, with regard to motor fluctuations, they found that the result was dependent on the adjusted results of one study (the UK-PDRG study) and if the unadjusted figures were used the overall result became insignificant. Additionally, results were not reported for a number of patients in these studies and a modified worst-case sensitivity analysis also made the results non-significant. (1++)

The meta-analysis[120] found more side effects were reported in:

- people with PD randomised to an MAOB inhibitor, treatment difference 1.36 (95% CI 1.02 to 1.80, p=0.04).

The Cochrane review[121] also found more adverse events with MAOB inhibitors; however, this was not a statistically significant difference. (1++)

The RCTs[132,133] found minimal or no side effects reported in either treatment group. (1++)

One meta-analysis[120] found more people in the MAOB inhibitor group withdrew due to adverse events than in the non-MAOB inhibitor group; treatment difference 2.16 (95% CI 1.44 to 3.23, p=0.0002). Similarly, the Cochrane review found significantly more withdrawals with MAOB inhibitors.[121] (1++)

One meta-analysis[120] found more deaths occurred in the MAOB inhibitor patients compared with controls but this was not a significant difference, while the Cochrane review[121] found a non-significant increase in deaths among patients treated with MAOB inhibitors compared with controls. (1++)

▷ From evidence to recommendation

The trial evidence supports the ability of MAOB inhibitors in PD to improve motor symptoms, improve activities of daily living and delay the need for levodopa. The evidence on them delaying motor complications is unclear. This is at the expense of more dopaminergic adverse events and, as a result, more withdrawals from treatment. There was no conclusive evidence of any increase in mortality on selegiline.

It is not possible from the evidence available to decide whether the lack of amphetamine metabolites with rasagiline confers any clinical benefit compared with selegiline.

RECOMMENDATION

R32   MAOB inhibitors may be used as a symptomatic treatment for people with early PD.   A

7.2.5 Beta-adrenergic antagonists (beta-blockers)

Beta-adrenergic antagonists (eg propanolol and oxprenolol) are well established in the treatment of the tremor seen in essential tremor and thyrotoxicosis.

Are beta-adrenergic antagonists effective in reducing the symptoms of PD?

▷ Methodology

A Cochrane systematic review[134] included four randomised controlled trials. Only 72 people with PD were included in these studies. All trials were randomised double-blind crossover studies.

Three of the crossover trials[135,136,137] in the systematic review did not present data from the end of the first arms. Since there is a carry-over risk, the systematic review did not analyse the data from these trials. One trial did report data from the first arm;[138] however, the trial did not state baseline scores, numbers of patients in each group, or standard deviations.

▷ Evidence statements

The systematic review was methodologically sound and hence it could technically be given a grading of 1++/1+. However, the methodological limitations of individual studies contained within the review meant that there were insufficient robust data from which to derive evidence statements.

The only evidence reported by the review was from a single trial[138] which found no significant difference between oxprenolol and placebo in mean total score for tremor.

Details of the data analysis were not given so it was not possible for the systematic review to determine whether the non-significance was based on comparison between the first and second arms (which could have been affected by a possible crossover effect) or between the therapy and placebo groups at the end of each arm.

▷ From evidence to recommendation

There is insufficient trial evidence for the efficacy or safety of beta-adrenergic antagonists in PD. However, the GDG felt that for selected people with PD with postural tremor they could be useful and safe.

RECOMMENDATION

R33   Beta-adrenergic antagonists may be used in the symptomatic treatment of selected
       people with postural tremor in PD, but should not be drugs of first choice.   D (GPP)

7.2.6 Amantadine

Amantadine was initially investigated as an anti-viral agent but found to be effective in PD by chance. The mechanism(s) of action of amantadine in PD are unclear.

What evidence is there to support the use of amantadine in early PD?

▷ Methodology

A Cochrane systematic review[139] was found which compared the effectiveness of amantadine versus placebo or levodopa in the treatment of people with early PD who are functionally disabled. The review included six studies, with a total sample size of 215 people with PD.

An additional randomised crossover trial[140] was found but excluded due to the following methodological limitations: methods of randomisation and allocation concealment not stated, limited patient characteristics given, no intention-to-treat analysis, and no power calculations provided for the small sample size (N=29).

Due to inadequate reporting of trial data, only two of the six trials within the systematic review had results that could be examined. However, in these two trials[141,142] only data for the trials' 'means' were given and thus no statistical analysis of the significance of the changes due to amantadine could be undertaken.

▷ Evidence statements

The systematic review was methodologically sound and hence it could technically be given a grading of 1++/1+. However, the methodological limitations of individual studies contained within the review meant that there were insufficient robust data from which to derive evidence statements.

▷ From evidence to recommendation

There are limited trial data to document the efficacy and safety of amantadine in early PD. This can be explained by its development in the 1970s, when trial design was in its infancy. The GDG concluded that, while amantadine should be available for the treatment of mild PD symptoms, other drug classes (ie levodopa, dopamine agonists) are more appropriate treatments for the early stages of the disease.

RECOMMENDATION

R34 Amantadine may be used as a treatment for people with early PD but should not be
a drug of first choice.   **D (GPP)**

7.2.7 Anticholinergics

Anticholinergics have been used to treat PD for over 100 years. They were introduced in the late 19th century after Charcot's work with hyoscine (scopolamine). In the mid-20th century, the selective centrally active muscarinic receptor antagonists were developed which had fewer peripheral side effects. These agents proliferated in the absence of more effective pharmaco-therapy, but the most commonly used for PD are trihexyphenidyl (benzhexol) and orphenadrine.

What is the evidence that selective muscarinic antagonists are effective and safe treatments for PD?

▷ Methodology

A Cochrane review[143] and an additional RCT[144] were found which addressed the effectiveness of anticholinergics in early PD.

One study[145] was excluded on the basis that the methodology did not constitute a randomised design between anticholinergic and levodopa treatment groups.

The Cochrane review included nine double-blind randomised crossover trials, with a total of 221 people. All of the trials compared the effectiveness of anticholinergics with placebo or no treatment. The RCT[144] was a single-blind study with a total of 82 people randomised to three groups: anticholinergics, levodopa and bromocriptine.

The Cochrane review authors highlighted that the outcome measures varied widely among the trials and the scales used to measure effectiveness were either the authors' own or no longer in current clinical use. The numerous methodological issues associated with these trials included: rating scales not being defined in detail, incomplete reporting of methodology and results, and heterogeneous study designs which precluded any analysis of the results.

▷ Evidence statements

The RCT[144] showed that the three anti-parkinsonian medications (anticholinergics, bromocriptine and levodopa) did not have qualitatively different effects upon various parkinsonian symptoms. The authors suggested that this may have been due to low level of disease severity. (1+)

The systematic review was methodologically sound and hence it could technically be given a grading of 1++/1+. However, the methodological limitations of individual studies contained within the review meant that there were insufficient robust data from which to derive evidence statements.

The authors of the review conclude that as monotherapy or as an adjunct to other anti-parkinsonian drugs, anticholinergics are more effective than placebo in improving motor function in PD in short-term use.

▷ From evidence to recommendation

There are insufficient data from RCTs on the efficacy and safety of anticholinergics in PD. This is particularly true of the claimed efficacy of this class in the treatment of tremor. However, the GDG concluded that anticholinergics should be available for the treatment of mild parkinsonian symptoms in people with no cognitive dysfunction. Their use should be regularly reviewed, but withdrawal can be difficult due to the re-emergence of motor impairments.

RECOMMENDATION

R35   Anticholinergics may be used as a symptomatic treatment typically in young people with early PD and severe tremor, but should not be drugs of first choice due to limited efficacy and the propensity to cause neuropsychiatric side effects.   **B**

7.3   Comparisons of drug classes

While proving the efficacy and safety of a drug class in placebo-controlled trials is important, particularly from the regulatory point of view, clinicians are keen to know how each class compares with others so that evidence-based treatment recommendations can be made for individual people. Such active comparator trials are rare in PD.

Recommendations will be presented at the end of this section for all drug comparisons.

7.3.1 Modified-release compared with immediate-release levodopa

It has been suggested that levodopa induces motor complications because of its short duration of action and thus the pulsatile stimulation of dopamine receptors. To avoid this, modified- or slow-release formulations of levodopa were developed.

What is the evidence that modified-release levodopa preparations delay the onset of motor complications?

▷ Methodology

Four studies[146–149] were found which addressed the effectiveness of modified-release levodopa compared with immediate-release levodopa in the treatment of early PD.

One study[146] was excluded due to lack of important information on drug dosages, randomisation methods, method of outcomes measurement and clinical criteria for the patient group. Another study was excluded as it was an open-trial design and therefore had increased potential for bias.[148]

One of the two included studies[147] examined the efficacy of immediate-release co-beneldopa (Madopar®; levodopa and benserazide) compared with modified-release (Madopar HBS/CR®), while the other study examined immediate-release co-careldopa (Sinemet®; levodopa and carbidopa) compared with modified-release (Sinemet CR®) formulation.[149]

▷ Evidence statements

With respect to clinical rating scales and quality of life:
- the co-careldopa study[149] (N=134) found:
  - ADL scores (UPDRS scale) were in favour of the modified-release preparation ($p=0.006$ year 1; $p=0.031$ year 5).
  - Nottingham Health Profile was in favour of modified-release for emotional reaction and social isolation ($p<0.05$). (1+)

Both studies[147,149] found no significant differences between the treatment groups for the following outcome measures of motor impairment:
- New York University Parkinson's Disease Scale (NYUPDS)
- Northwestern University Disability Scale (NUDS)
- UPDRS
- Hoehn and Yahr scales
- Schwab and England scores. (1+)

One study[149] reported no significant difference between treatment groups for motor fluctuations (primary endpoint) either by diary data or by questionnaire. With respect to drug dosage, this study[149] (N=618) found the average number of daily doses was in favour of the modified-release preparation ($p<0.005$), while the other study[147] found no differences. (1+)

With respect to adverse effects, one study[147] reported no significant differences between the two groups. (1+)

With respect to withdrawal rates, one study[149] found the number of withdrawals was higher in the immediate-release group (p=0.007). (1+)

▷ From evidence to recommendation

This evidence suggests that there is no value in using the existing modified-release levodopa preparations to delay the onset of motor complications.

RECOMMENDATION

R36   Modified-release levodopa preparations should not be used to delay the onset of motor complications in people with early PD.   A

7.3.2 Dopamine agonists compared with levodopa

How effective and safe are dopamine agonists compared with levodopa in the treatment of functionally disabled early PD?

▷ Methodology

Twelve RCTs[42,116,118,150–158] were found which addressed whether dopamine agonists were more effective than levodopa in treating people with early PD who are functionally disabled.

Eight of these papers were randomised double-blind studies.[116,118,150–153,155,158] One of these studies[154] was single blind and three were open-trial designs.[42,156,157] Two of the papers[116,153] included were by the same group of investigators; the more recent publication[116] reported 10-year follow-up outcomes for the same cohort of people.

The sample sizes ranged from 18 to 782 (median 82) and the trial durations ranged from 5.8 months to 120 months (median 44.4 months or 3.7 years).

▷ Evidence statements

The results from the eight trials are summarised in Table 7.2.

Table 7.2 Dopamine agonist (DA) compared with levodopa (LD) treatment (1+)	
Outcome	**DA versus LD**
Quality of Life (PDQUALIF and EuroQol scores)	NS[158]
UPDRS total	NS[150] PPX[158]
UPDRS motor (III)	NS[151] PPX[158], RP[152]
UPDRS ADL (II)	NS[152,118] PPX[158]
Hoehn and Yahr	NS[153,154]
Columbia Score	NS[151,155] BR[153]

continued

Table 7.2 Dopamine agonist (DA) compared with levodopa (LD) treatment (1+) – *continued*	
Outcome	**DA versus LD**
NUDS	NS[155] BR[153]
Webster scale	NS[154] BR[42]
Risk of developing motor complications	CB[118], BR[156], PPX[158]
Risk of dyskinesias	NS[118,151,155], BR[42,152,153,156], PPX[158], RP[152], BR[153], BR[42]
Risk of wearing-off	NS[151,155] PPX[158]
Risk of dystonia	NS[151,158] BR[153]
Need for supplemental levodopa	PPX[158]
Adverse events (all)	NS[118,150–152,154–156]
Somnolence, oedema, hallucinations	PPX[158]
Mortality	NS[156] BR[42]
Withdrawals	NS [118,150-152,154,157]

PPX = pramipexole; RP = ropinirole; BR = bromocriptine; CB = cabergoline; PPX/RP/BR/CB = in favour (p<0.05) of dopamine agonist treatment; LD = in favour (p<0.05) of levodopa treatment; NS = non-significant difference between treatment groups.

7.3.3 Dopamine agonists plus levodopa compared with levodopa

What is the effectiveness of dopamine agonists plus levodopa compared with levodopa monotherapy in the treatment of functionally disabled early PD?

▷ Methodology

Eight papers[115,151,154,157,159–162] were found which addressed the effectiveness of dopamine agonists combined with levodopa compared with levodopa monotherapy. Five of these studies[115,151,154,160,161] were included in a Cochrane review,[163] but these papers were reviewed independently for additional outcomes and follow-up studies.

Five of the trials[115,157,159,160,162] were open label for the majority of the follow-up, one trial[154] was single blind and one trial[151] was double blind.

The sample size ranged from 20 to 587 people (median 78) and the trial duration ranged from 12 months to 5 years.

Five articles were appraised (see Table 7.3) and met quality criteria.[164–168] No UK studies were identified.

Table 7.3 Dopamine plus levodopa compared with levodopa monotherapy (1+)	
Outcome	**Significance**
Clinical rating scales	
UPDRS total	NS[157]
UPDRS II (activities of daily living)	NS[151,160] Li/LD[159]
UPDRS III (motor)	Li/LD[159,161], BR/LD[161]
UPDRS IV	NS[159,161]
UPDRS addendum (motor complications) scores	Li/LD[159]
On time during day	NS[161]
Hoehn and Yahr	NS[154,159,160,162] LD[161]
Webster score	NS[154] BR/LD[161]
Columbia University Rating Scale (CURS)	BR/LD[161]
Modified CURS	NS[151]
Schwab and England score	Li/LD[159]
NUDS	LD[161]
Adverse events	
All events	NS[151,154]
Mortality	BR/LD[115]
Nausea/vomiting	LD[161]
Fatigue/weakness	LD[161]
Hallucinations/confusion	LD[161]
Withdrawal rates	
Number of drop-outs	NS[151,154,157] Li/LD[159]

LD = levodopa; Li = lisuride; BR = bromocriptine; LD = in favour (p<0.05) of levodopa monotherapy; Li or BR/LD = in favour of (p<0.05) combination therapy; NS = non-significant.

▷ Health economic methodology

A US study assessed the cost-effectiveness of pramipexole compared with no pramipexole in early PD by estimating the cost per quality-adjusted life year (QALY) during a life-time horizon.[164]

One study estimated the incremental cost (IC) per QALY of initial pramipexole treatment compared with initial levodopa treatment in early PD based on a 4-year US and Canadian multi-centre RCT.[169]

A Canadian study derived the costs per day per patient to substitute levodopa plus benserazide by ropinirole over a 5-year time horizon in a cost-minimisation analysis.[166]

A German study evaluated cabergoline compared with levodopa monotherapy by estimating the cost per decreased UPDRS score based on a Markov model with a 10-year time horizon and the ICs per additional motor complication-free patient.[167]

A Swedish study evaluated the cost-effectiveness of early cabergoline treatment compared with levodopa in the early treatment of PD by estimating the cost per year of motor complications over 5 years.[168]

A cost-minimisation analysis of dopamine agonist compared with levodopa in initial PD therapy was estimated from the perspective of the NHS over a 1-year period (Appendix E).

▷ Health economic evidence statements

In people with early PD, the incremental cost-effectiveness for pramipexole compared with no pramipexole is $8,840 in US$ 1997 (approximately £5,510) per QALY from a societal perspective and $34,420 (approximately £21,480) per QALY without including productivity gains from pramipexole.[164] However, cost-effectiveness results were sensitive to changes in the model's parameters, resulting in cost per QALYs of $3,880 (approximately £2,420) when direct medical costs are 50% higher, $46,470 (approximately £28,990) when the rate of change of UPDRS after levodopa is 0.5 (versus 1.375 baseline) and $908,310 (approximately £566,720) when no-pramipexole treatment includes pergolide as adjunct.

One study estimated the incremental cost-effectiveness of initial pramipexole treatment compared with initial levodopa treatment in patients with early PD over a 4-year time period. The incremental cost-effectiveness ratio for pramipexole was $43,000 in US$ (approximately £24,700) per QALY, using the EQ-5D health-related quality of life measure. However, the pramipexole strategy is dominated by the levodopa strategy when using the EQ-VAS to derive the health utilities.[165]

Assuming equivalent clinical effectiveness, the cost of replacing levodopa plus benserazide with ropinirole in a Canadian setting gives a net IC of $4.14 (£2.38) per patient day. From a societal perspective, productivity and caregiver utilisation savings offset the drug acquisition cost for ropinirole. Varying the key parameters (nursing home admission rates, cost of caregiver time and proportion of people with disabling dyskinesias who lost their jobs) by 15–20%, did not change the direction of the results.[166]

In people aged 60 years or over, cabergoline monotherapy was estimated to cost approximately an additional €1,030 in Euro 2002 (approximately £718) per unit decrease in UPDRS score. This value was robust to changes in the discount rate, cost data and mortality assessed in the sensitivity analysis. Levodopa monotherapy dominated cabergoline monotherapy in people under 60 years of age. Incremental costs per additional motor complication-free patient were estimated at €104,400 (approximately £72,710) in people under 60 years of age and €57,900 (approximately £40,330) in people aged 60 years or over based on subsamples of the clinical trial used for data analysis.[167]

One study estimated an incremental cost-effectiveness of €13,860 (approximately £9,660) per year of motor complications avoided with cabergoline treatment.[168]

The baseline estimates result in an IC of £2,390 for pramipexole treatment over a 1-year period. The unit cost of pramipexole had the most impact on the ICs and resulted in the widest range of all the IC estimates (£1,880 to £2,640). On the basis of equivalent quality of life between the treatments, the levodopa strategy is the less costly option (see Appendix E).

▷ From evidence to recommendation

There is a wealth of evidence from dopamine agonist compared with levodopa trials that agonists delay the onset of motor complications. However, there is some evidence that levodopa treats motor impairments and disability better. Agonists also lead to more adverse events such as somnolence, oedema and hallucinations, but this does not lead to an excess of withdrawals from the trials.

It is more difficult to interpret the generally older dopamine agonist combined with levodopa compared with levodopa monotherapy trials. There is some suggestion of combination therapy treating motor impairments and disability better than levodopa but at the expense of more adverse events such as nausea, vomiting, fatigue, hallucinations and confusion. There are few data on motor complications.

The implication is that to delay motor complications, dopamine agonists should be used initially without levodopa. However, patients' motor function will not be treated as well and they may suffer more side effects. This issue requires further clarification in trials using patient-rated quality of life as the primary outcome measure. The GDG acknowledged that the ongoing PD MED trial might provide additional data on the cost benefits of the various agents. Although useful for economic evaluations, the EQ-5D is a relatively insensitive measure of health-related quality of life. Given that no difference was detected in the PDQUALIF or EQ-VAS scales, the GDG concluded that there was no clear evidence of a clinically important difference in overall quality of life between the two treatment strategies (see Appendix E). This assumption was used in the economic model that indicated the levodopa strategy is the less costly short-term option.

7.3.4 Monoamine oxidase type B inhibitors compared with levodopa

How effective are MAOB inhibitors compared with levodopa in managing people with early PD?

▷ Methodology

Two meta-analyses[120,121] and a randomised crossover trial[133] which addressed the effectiveness of MAOB inhibitors in treating people with early PD were included.

The meta-analyses[120,121] compared MAOBs with controls (and did not differentiate between levodopa and placebo controls). In many of the included trials, the MAOB inhibitors were not given alone but were in combination with levodopa therapy. The RCT[133] also compared people on levodopa plus selegiline with levodopa plus placebo.

One meta-analysis[120] included 3,525 people with PD from 17 randomised trials while the other (a Cochrane review) included 2,422 people with PD from 10 trials.[121] The randomised crossover trial consisted of 15 people with PD. The small sample size may have underpowered the study and could be reflective of the non-significant results, when compared with the large meta-analysis.

▷ Evidence statements

With respect to clinical rating scales:

- Only one study[42] in the meta-analyses[120,121] reported mean Webster disability scores. The trial reported that the difference was non-significant between groups on levodopa plus selegiline compared with levodopa alone (no p values given). (1+)
- The randomised crossover trial[133] reported no significant differences between scores for the Webster rating scale (total scores) in people with PD on levodopa plus selegiline compared with levodopa alone. (1++)

With respect to motor complications, only one study[156] from one meta-analysis[120] reported the following:

- Motor fluctuations were more frequent among levodopa-treated people (29.7%) than selegiline-treated people (18.7%).
- People assigned to selegiline were significantly less likely to experience motor fluctuations (non-significant, no p value stated).
- Dyskinesias occurred less frequently in the selegiline group (20.7%) than the levodopa group (27.1%). (1+)

With respect to need for levodopa therapy, the combined trials in the meta-analysis[120] found:

- The dose of levodopa required for adequate symptom control was 67 mg lower in the selegiline arm (95% CI 14 to 119, p=0.01).
- All studies showed higher levodopa doses in the control groups than in patients treated with MAOB inhibitors (meta-analysis not performed for this outcome).[121] (1+)

With respect to withdrawal rates:

- Only one study[156] from one meta-analysis[120] reported data on withdrawal rates. The trial found the probability of people ceasing treatment in the selegiline group was about threefold higher than in those assigned to levodopa.
- Most of these withdrawals occurred after the first 6 months and were due to peoples' or physicians' determination of inefficacy (two people stopped because of sleep disturbance side effects). (1+)

With respect to mortality:

- One study[42] in the meta-analyses[120,121] reported the following between levodopa monotherapy and levodopa plus selegiline therapy:
  - for all deaths, unadjusted hazard ratio of 1.22 (95% CI 0.95 to 1.55, no p value stated)
  - first 5 years of study, unadjusted hazard ratio of 1.41 (95% CI 0.92 to 2.17, p=0.27).
- Another study[156] in one meta-analysis found no difference between rates of mortality. (1+)

▷ From evidence to recommendation

Selegiline delays the onset of motor complications and the need for levodopa but at the expense of more withdrawals due to lack of efficacy. There are few trial data on selegiline's effect on motor impairments and none on quality of life. The clinical experience of the GDG suggests that selegiline is less effective than levodopa in the treatment of functional impairments and disability in PD. There are no trial data or clinical experience on the comparative efficacy and safety of rasagiline. Further trials to compare MAOB therapy with levodopa are required.

7.3.5 Monoamine oxidase type B inhibitors compared with dopamine agonists

How effective are MAOB inhibitors compared with dopamine agonists in the treatment of early PD?

▷ Methodology

Only two RCTs[156,42] were found which compared the effectiveness of MAOB inhibitors and dopamine agonists in the treatment of early PD.

Both studies included a third levodopa therapy arm. Most of the disability and motor function analysis in the UK-PDRG study[42] involved the comparison of bromocriptine with levodopa. Similarly, the other trial[156] used the levodopa group as the reference group and did not provide statistical analysis of the results for the comparison of selegiline and dopamine agonists.

The UK-PDRG study[42] consisted of 782 people with PD, and compared the effectiveness of levodopa, levodopa and selegiline and bromocriptine. The other study[156] consisted of 473 people with PD, and compared the effectiveness of selegiline, levodopa and dopamine agonists (bromocriptine and lisuride). It is important to note that selegiline in the UK-PDRG trial[42] was combined with levodopa therapy, whereas the other study[156] used selegiline as a monotherapy (levodopa could be added if physician deemed selegiline alone to be ineffective).

▷ Evidence statements

In the UK-PDRG study,[42] after 9 years of follow-up, there was a non-significant difference in Webster scores (adjusted for baseline score) between the bromocriptine group and the levodopa plus selegiline group. (1+)

With respect to motor complications, one study[156] found no significant differences in:
- motor fluctuations
- mean time to motor fluctuation
- frequency of dyskinesias
- difference in time to dyskinesia between dopamine agonist and MAOB inhibitor groups. (1+)

With respect to mortality, the UK-PDRG study[42] found non-significant differences in mortality between levodopa plus selegiline and bromocriptine groups:
- unadjusted hazard ratio for overall deaths (non-significant)
- unadjusted hazard ratio in first 5 years was (p=0.27). (1+)

The other study[156] found no significant difference in mortality between the dopamine agonist groups and the selegiline group. (1+)

With respect to withdrawal rates, one study[156] reported the following.

- Most people with PD withdrew from dopamine agonists because of nausea/vomiting or postural hypotension or both (43/53 people).
- Most of the withdrawals in the selegiline group occurred in the first 6 months of treatment and were due to lack of efficacy.
- Combination therapy was started in 40.7% of people on dopamine agonists and 63.9% of people on selegiline.
- The initiation of levodopa therapy was delayed for a median of 30 months in dopamine agonist group and 15 months in selegiline group. (1+)

▷ From evidence to recommendation

While there was no difference in the delaying of motor complications between MAOB inhibitors and dopamine agonists, there is a suggestion that agonists are more effective than MAOB inhibitors in delaying the need for levodopa. More people with PD withdraw from MAOB inhibitors because of lack of efficacy; however, this evidence is based on just two studies and all of the data relates to selegiline.

7.4 Choice of initial pharmacological therapy in early Parkinson's disease

7.4.1 From evidence to recommendation

See Table 7.1 for a summary of the drugs covered within this section.

It was evident from reviewing the evidence base that there is no single drug of choice in the initial pharmacotherapy of early PD.

Further trials are required to compare the initial treatment of PD with levodopa, dopamine agonists and MAOB inhibitors, preferably using quality-of-life and health economics outcome measures. The UK PD MED trial will attempt to address these comparisons. More information can be found from **www.pdmed.bham.ac.uk**

RECOMMENDATION

R37   It is not possible to identify a universal first-choice drug therapy for people with early PD. The choice of drug first prescribed should take into account:

- clinical and lifestyle characteristics
- patient preference, after the patient has been informed of the short- and long-term benefits and drawbacks of the drug classes.   **D (GPP)**

7.5 Later pharmacological therapy

'"Off" is unmedicated. At my stage, it can get to where I can't really speak that well and I can't inflect. I can't really use my face. I'll be shaking. And that's "off". And then "on" is a version of this, which is when the medication's working. I have "on" plus, because I have a little bit of dyskinesia, which is a function of the medication.'

(patient)[3]

7.5.1 Introduction

It was evident from reviewing the evidence base that there is no single drug of choice in the pharmacotherapy of later PD. Table 7.4 may help to guide the reader through the following section.

			Possible risk of side effects	
Table 7.4 Options for adjuvant pharmacotherapy in later PD				
Adjuvant therapy for later PD	**First-choice option**	**Symptom control**	**Motor complications**	**Other adverse events**
Dopamine agonists	✓	++	↓	↑
COMT inhibitors	✓	++	↓	↑
MAOB inhibitors	✓	++	↓	↑
Amantadine	✗	NS	↓	↑
Apomorphine	✗	+	↓	↑

+++ = Good degree of symptom control.
++ = Moderate degree of symptom control.
+ = Limited degree of symptom control.
↑ = Evidence of increased motor complications/other adverse events.
↓ = Evidence of reduced motor complications/other adverse events.
NS = Non-significant result.

7.5.2 Levodopa

Since most people with PD will eventually need levodopa, they will all with time develop motor complications. While the latter can be mild and not interfere with a person's quality of life, for some they can be severely incapacitating. Adjuvant drugs to take with levodopa have been developed with the aim of reducing these complications and improving quality of life.

The previous section contains a statement about the methodological limitations of symptomatic therapy studies and recommendations about symptomatic pharmacological therapies for both early and later disease.

The GDG was concerned that the old practice of withdrawing PD patients from medication in the hope of improving motor complications is dangerous. Such 'drug holidays' can lead to severe immobility with secondary chest infection, neuroleptic malignant syndrome and death. This practice is rarely performed now and, because of the dangers, it should be abandoned.

▷ Modified-release levodopa

Wearing off of the effects of levodopa and peak dose dyskinesia is largely caused by pulsatile stimulation of dopamine receptors, which is related to the intermittent administration of exogenous immediate-release levodopa. One potential way to overcome this is to prolong the effect of each dose of levodopa by administering controlled or modified-release levodopa preparations. Such preparations of co-careldopa (Sinemet CR®) and co-beneldopa (Madopar HBS/CR®) have been developed.

Can modified-release preparations of levodopa reduce motor complications compared with immediate-release preparations?

▷ Methodology

Eleven randomised controlled trials[170–180] comparing the effect of controlled-release 50/500 mg levodopa with immediate-release 25/100 levodopa in later PD were found. The sample size (range 19–202, mean 57) and mean age of people (range 58–67 years, mean 62.8) varied between trials.

Most of the included studies[170–178,180] used the co-careldopa formulation of either 25/100 or 50/200 for the immediate-release and controlled-release tablets, respectively. Only one trial[179] used 25/200 for the immediate-release dosage, but administered 50/200 for controlled release. None of the included trials used the co-beneldopa formulation.

Only one trial reported a washout period between trials[179] all other trials analysed data from either the end of the trial arms or at week 2 or later in each arm.

All of the included trials started with an open-label titration phase in which the optimal anti-parkinsonian dose and inter-dose interval for each treatment were determined. In many of the trials a large percentage of people withdrew (35%,[179] 31%,[175] 26%,[170] 24%,[173] 18%,[180] 17%[171]) during the open phase because of inconsistencies with response, delayed onset of drug action or adverse events. Due to the already small sample size (average 60), lack of power calculations and intention-to-treat analysis, these studies were highly biased towards a pre-selected patient population. The trial duration was also very short with a range of 8–24 weeks.

▷ Evidence statements

The results of the trials are summarised in Table 7.5.

With respect to adverse events:
- Most common adverse events for both treatments included dizziness, dyskinesia, dystonia, headache, hallucinations, nausea, vomiting, hypotension and confusion.[171,176,177]
- There was no significant difference in the reported incidence of adverse events between the two treatment groups.[171,174,180]
- One study[177] reported people treated with controlled-release levodopa had a higher incidence of self-reported adverse events ($p<0.05$) but not a higher frequency. (1+)

Table 7.5 Controlled-release compared with immediate-release levodopa	
Outcome measures	Results
Total number of trials	11
Total sample size (N)	646
Clinical rating scales	
UPDRS motor score	CR[173]
Hoehn and Yahr score	CR[175]
NYUPDS score (after 6 months' treatment)	CR[177]
SEALD score	CR[171]
Patient-rated global improvement	CR[175]
Physician-rated global improvement	CR[175]
Patient-reported helpfulness of medication and improvement in clinical fluctuations	CR[171]
Motor complications	
On time	CR[173,175,178,179] IR[173]
Off time	CR[173,177,179]
Dyskinesia duration	IR[178]
Levodopa dose	
Mean doses per day	CR[170,172,173,175,180] NS[177]
Mean interdose interval	CR[170,173,180]
Mean daily levodopa dose (mg/d)	IR[171–174,176,178–181]

CR = controlled release - favouring (p<0.05) CR; IR = immediate release - favouring (p<0.05) IR; NS = non-significant (p>0.05).

With respect to withdrawal rates:

- Two studies[171,172] found 52–54% of people preferred controlled release over 27–33% of people who preferred immediate release.
- Two studies found high numbers of people continuing controlled-release therapy after the completion of their trials (100%[179] and 87%[180]).
- Common reasons for withdrawal include adverse events, insufficient therapeutic response, lack of compliance and missing follow-up appointments.[176,177] (1+)

▷ From evidence to recommendation

The trial evidence suggests that modified-release levodopa preparations can satisfactorily reduce motor fluctuations. However, the GDG had considerable reservations about the design of many of the trials. Subsequent clinical practice has found that switching directly from immediate- to modified-release levodopa leads to an increase in off time. This is probably due to poorer absorption of modified-release preparations from the gut. As a result, modified-release levodopa is rarely used to manage motor complications. Modified-release preparations are also more expensive than immediate-release formulations. The GDG concluded that combinations of modified- and immediate-release levodopa could be useful in a small number of people with motor complications.

RECOMMENDATION

R38   Modified-release levodopa preparations may be used to reduce motor complications in
       people with later PD but should not be drugs of first choice.   B

7.5.3   Dopamine agonists

While recent trial work has concentrated on the use of dopamine agonists as initial therapy in PD, these agents were originally introduced as adjuvant therapy to reduce motor complications in later disease.

How effective and safe are dopamine agonists as adjuvant therapy in later PD?

▷   Methodology

Nine papers, which included six Cochrane reviews[182–187] and three additional RCTs,[188–190] were found that addressed the effectiveness of adding dopamine agonists compared with placebo in the treatment of motor complications in people with later PD. Sample sizes of these trials are listed in Table 7.6. No RCTs were found on lisuride's effectiveness.

There were several issues for consideration with the trials included in the Cochrane reviews,[182–187] such as:
- inclusion of phase II and III studies and unpublished papers
- additional unpublished data obtained from investigators or manufacturers sought by the Cochrane authors.

The three RCTs[188–190] that were published since the Cochrane reviews were well designed and had sound methodologies.

▷   Evidence statements

With respect to quality of life:
- two trials, one[191] included in the Cochrane review[186] and another published after the review,[188] reported the following outcomes in favour of pramipexole:
    - Functional Status Questionnaire Basic ADL
    - mental health scales
    - EuroQol Scale
    - patient diaries (impairment of daily living and severity of tremor ($p<0.0001$). (1++)

With respect to clinical rating scales, motor complications and levodopa dose reduction, improvement was found to be in favour of the dopamine agonists (bromocriptine, cabergoline, pergolide, pramipexole and ropinirole) in most of the included trials (Table 7.6).

Table 7.6 Dopamine agonists compared with placebo in later PD

	Bromocriptine 182(192–198)	Cabergoline 183(199–201)	Pergolide 185(202)	Pramipexole 186(191,203–205),188–190	Ropinirole 187(206–208)
Number of trials	7	3	1	7	3
Sample size (N)	400	268	376	1,228	263
Clinical rating scales					
UPDRS II	–	DA[201] NS[199]	–	DA[191,203–205,189,190]	–
UPDRS III	–	DA[201] NS[199]	–	DA[191,203,204,189,190] NS[205]	–
UPDRS IV	–	–	–	DA[203,204] P NS[191,205]	–
Hoehn and Yahr	–	NS[200,201]	DA[202]	DA[203] NS[191]	–
S & E	–	NS[199,200]	–	A[203] NS[191]	–
MCRS*	–	–	DA[202]	–	–
Global rating					
Clinician	–	DA[200]	–	DA[204,188,190]	DA
Motor complications					
Dyskinesia	LD[198]	–	LD[202]	–	LD[207]
Off time	NS[195,197]	NS[199,200]	DA[202]	DA[191,203–205,189]	DA[207]
Impairment	DA[195,196] NS[198]	–	–	–	DA[207]
Wearing-off	DA[196]	–	–	–	–
Levodopa					
Levodopa dose reduction	NS[196]	DA[201]	DA[202]	DA[191,203,205]	DA[207]
Adverse events					
Hallucinations	–	NS[199–201]	P[202]	P[191,203,204]	–
Dyskinesia	–	NS[199]	P[202]	DA[191,203,204]	P[207]
Hypotension	NS	DA[199–201]	–	NS[191,203–205]	–
Withdrawal rate					
All cause	NS	NS[199–201]	NS[202]	DA[191,203]	NS[207]
Adverse events	–	–	P[202]	–	–

DA = favouring dopamine agonist (p<0.05); P = favouring placebo (p<0.05); – = not reported; NS = non-significant (p>0.05).
References for papers included in Cochrane reviews.
*Modified Columbia Rating Scale including gait, tremor, ADL and motor scores.

▷ From evidence to recommendation

In people with PD and motor complications, adjuvant dopamine agonist therapy reduces off time and levodopa dose and improves motor impairments and activities of daily living. This is at the expense of increased dopaminergic adverse events including dyskinesia, hallucinations and postural hypotension. These conclusions are based on short-term trials and the long-term acceptability of adjuvant agonist therapy remains to be evaluated.

Concerns regarding serosal reactions with ergot-derived dopamine agonists have been considered earlier in this chapter.

RECOMMENDATIONS

R39   Dopamine agonists may be used to reduce motor fluctuations in people with later PD.   **A**

R40   If an ergot-derived dopamine agonist is used, the patient should have a minimum of renal function tests, ESR and chest radiograph performed before starting treatment and annually thereafter.*   **D (GPP)**

R41   A dopamine agonist should be titrated to a clinically efficacious dose. If side effects prevent this, then another agonist or a drug from another class should be used in its place.   **D (GPP)**

R42   In view of the monitoring required with ergot-derived dopamine agonists, a non-ergot-derived agonist should be preferred in most cases.   **D (GPP)**

7.5.4 Monoamine oxidase type B inhibitors

The MAOB inhibitor selegiline was first used as a symptomatic treatment for PD before it was evaluated as a possible neuroprotective therapy (Chapter 6). More recently, rasagiline has become available as another MAOB inhibitor with symptomatic effects in PD.

How effective and safe are these MAOB inhibitors in treating the motor complications of later PD?

▷ Methodology

Ten randomised double-blind placebo-controlled trials[209–218] were found which addressed the effectiveness of MAOB inhibitors as an adjunct to levodopa treatment in people with later PD and motor complications. Of these nine trials, six were parallel group studies and three were crossover trials.

All of the trials apart from three,[209,217,218] investigated the effectiveness of conventional selegiline treatment. Two RCTs[217,218] investigated the effectiveness of rasagiline, while the other[209] assessed the effectiveness of Zelapar® selegiline, a formulation that dissolves on contact with saliva and undergoes pregastric absorption.

---

*Full details of the restrictions on pergolide use and monitoring are available in the Summary of Product Characteristics.

A common methodological issue in all the conventional selegiline trials was the lack of sample size calculations. Most of these trials failed to demonstrate a significant difference in many of the outcomes measures investigated between active treatment and placebo. The small sample sizes (range 19–96, mean 54.6) and the short-term duration (range 3–8 weeks, mean 6.7 weeks) need to be taken into consideration.

One large (N=687) RCT (LARGO)[217] compared rasagiline with entacapone and placebo over 18 weeks. Another RCT (PRESTO)[218] with a large sample size (N=472) and duration of 26 weeks compared two different doses of rasagiline (0.5 or 1 mg) with placebo.

The Zelapar® selegiline study[209] was a (N=140) study of 12 weeks' duration. The only shortcoming of this trial was the lack of a conventional selegiline arm to directly compare the two formulations.

Most of the studies using conventional selegiline used a dose of 10 mg/day. One study[214] used a dosing sequence of 0–5–10 mg/day in a random order, another study[211] started with 5 mg/day in the first 4 weeks and increased to 10 mg/day for the final 4 weeks, and only one study[210] used 5 mg/day for the entire trial duration of 8 weeks. The rasagiline study administered a dose of 1 mg/day for 18 weeks. The study on Zelapar® selegiline used a dose of 1.25–2.5 mg/day for 12 weeks.

▷ Evidence statements

Outcomes that favoured (p<0.05) conventional selegiline were:
- Physician preference[211]
- Webster Rating Scale[211]
- Modified Columbia Rating Scale: 5/22 items (dressing, dysarthria, hypomimia, sialorrhoea, tremor)[212]
- Disability Scale: 2/22 items (facial expression and resting tremor)[213]
- Investigator's Global Subjective Opinion: more likely to have experienced improvement than worsened or no change.[213] (1+)

With respect to patient observations of conventional selegiline:
- At the end of the 6-week treatment period 76% of people reported themselves to be improved in the selegiline group and only 26% in the placebo group.[212]
- People reported the following while on selegiline treatment: dose of levodopa lasted longer, transitions between on and off periods were less abrupt, on periods were better, off periods were less severe.[216] (1+)

With respect to long-term follow-up:
- One study[215] performed a long-term blinded follow-up. People selected the treatment period they preferred during the randomised short-term trial and they were maintained on that preferred treatment for about 16 months on average. The follow-up study found:
  - The average levodopa dose was significantly lower (p<0.001) in selegiline-treated people.
  - The average dosing frequency was also lower in the selegiline group (p<0.01). (2+)

Table 7.7 MAOB inhibitor compared with placebo

Outcome	Conventional selegiline	Rasagiline	Zelapar® selegiline
Number of trials	7	2	1
Sample size (N)	169	1,159	140
Quality of life			
PDQUALIF scores	–	NS[218]	–
Clinical rating scales			
UPDRS total	–	R[217]	–
UPDRS motor (on)	–	R[217,218]	–
UPDRS ADL (off)	–	R[217,218]	–
UPDRS subscores	–	R[217,218]	–
Schwab and England ADL	–	R[218]	–
Patient diaries: proportion of people with improvement	SEL[212,213]	–	–
Clinician Global Impression Scale	–	R[217,218]	SEL[209]
Patient Global Impression Scale	–	–	SEL[209]
Motor complications			
On-off episodes	SEL[210]	–	–
On time	SEL[214]	R[217,218]	SEL[209]
Off time	SEL[214]	R[217,218]	SEL[209]
On time with dyskinesia (increased)	P[214]	NS[217] R[218]	–
Tremor	SEL[215]	R[217]	–
Daily levodopa dose			
Levodopa dose reduction	SEL[211,215,216]	R[217]	–
Adverse events and withdrawal rates			
Any adverse events	NS	NS[217]	NS[209]
All-cause withdrawal rates	NS	NS[217,218]	NS[209]

SEL = favouring selegiline (p<0.05); R = favouring rasagiline (p<0.05); P = favouring placebo (p<0.05); – = not reported; NS = non-significant (p>0.05).

One rasagiline RCT[218] reported a significant (p<0.05) increase in adverse events in the treatment group:

- Dyskinesias were reported as an adverse event by 10% receiving placebo and by 18% receiving either dose of rasagiline.
- Weight loss, vomiting and anorexia were reported in 1.0 mg/day group.
- Balance difficulty and depression were reported in 0.5 mg/day group. (1++)

▷ From evidence to recommendation

The size and quality of the adjuvant selegiline trials was poor, so it is impossible to reach firm conclusions about its efficacy and safety in later PD. The more recent study with the buccal formulation of selegiline and two large oral rasagiline trials provide more convincing evidence for the efficacy and safety of MAOB inhibitors in later PD. However, all studies were of short duration, so no comments on the long-term benefits and drawbacks of these agents can be made.

RECOMMENDATION

R43   MAOB inhibitors may be used to reduce motor fluctuations in people with later PD.   **A**

7.5.5   Catechol-O-methyl transferase inhibitors

Levodopa is now always combined with carbidopa (co-careldopa) or benserazide (co-beneldopa) to block its metabolism by dopa decarboxylase. This increases levodopa bioavailability by twofold to threefold and reduces peripheral side effects. However, only 5–10% of each levodopa dose crosses the blood-brain barrier, the rest being metabolised to 3-O-methyldopa by catechol-O-methyl transferase (COMT). The aim of COMT inhibitors is to further reduce the metabolism of levodopa and thus increase the amount crossing into the brain.

Two COMT inhibitors are available: entacapone and tolcapone. These lead to a 30–50% increase in levodopa half-life and a 25–100% increase in the levodopa concentration versus time curve (area under the curve); they do not increase the maximum plasma concentration of levodopa.[219] Most of this occurs because of peripheral inhibition, but tolcapone also has a central effect in the brain.

Tolcapone was the first COMT inhibitor to enter clinical practice in England and Wales but its European product licence was withdrawn in November 1998 after three cases of fatal hepatic toxicity. However, after further clinical experience in other markets and a forced switch from entacapone to tolcapone study, it has recently been reintroduced in Europe. It is currently licensed, at a dose of 100 mg three times per day, for people who have failed on entacapone, and requires mandatory liver function test monitoring at 2-week intervals for the first year of treatment followed by less stringent monitoring ad infinitum.

Entacapone has been combined with the levodopa plus carbidopa combination (co-careldopa) as a triple combination called Stalevo®. One study has shown that Stalevo® simplifies the taking of medication, which is more acceptable to patients.[220]

How effective are these COMT inhibitors in reducing the motor complications of later PD?

▷ Methodology

A Cochrane review[221] was found which addressed the effectiveness of the COMT inhibitors tolcapone and entacapone compared with placebo in people with PD suffering from motor complications.

Two additional RCTs[217,222] were found after the Cochrane search date. One RCT[217] compared entacapone (200 mg) with placebo (LARGO). The study[217] had a large (N=456) sample size and a trial duration of 18 weeks. The other RCT[222] compared entacapone (200 mg) with levodopa monotherapy. The study sample size was large (N=270) and the trial duration was 13 weeks. The methodological limitations of this study were lack of reported methods of randomisation and allocation concealment.

An additional RCT[223] was also found but excluded on the basis of patient characteristics. The people included in this trial could not experience end-of-dose wearing off within 4 hours of levodopa use, and had an average disease duration of 4.5 years. The results of this trial were not included due to the absence of motor complications.

The Cochrane review consisted of 14 trials (13 phase III, one phase II) and 2,566 patents with PD and motor fluctuations. Eight trials[224–231] examined entacapone compared with placebo (N=1560) and six trials[232–237] examined tolcapone compared with placebo (N=1006). Two of the included entacapone papers[229,230] were abstracts; however, the results were consistent with the full publications. The level of evidence for the Cochrane review is graded as 1++, which is based on the review's methodology and not that of the individual trials.

Issues for consideration with the Cochrane entacapone studies included: lack of randomisation and allocation concealment methods, lack of methodological detail available from the abstracts, and two studies did not state the method of data analysis. In addition, one of the entacapone studies[228] was a crossover design (N=26) without a washout period, and the results were presented as a combination of the two trial arms. The review did not use the results of this study in the meta-analysis.

▷ Evidence statements

Table 7.8 summarises the evidence for the effectiveness of COMT inhibitors compared with placebo.

The additional RCT[222] which compared entacapone with levodopa monotherapy reported the following significant (p<0.05) results in favour of combined therapy:
- improvement in UPDRS II (ADL) score, treatment difference –1.6 (95% CI –2.4 to –0.8, p=0.0001)
- UPDRS III (motor) scores decreased, treatment difference –1.9 (95% CI –3.7 to –0.2, p=0.03)
- mean UPDRS total score decreased, treatment difference –3.6 (95% CI –6.0 to –1.2, p=0.004)
- fluctuation sum score (UPDRS IVb) decreased, treatment difference –0.3 (95% CI –0.5 to –0.1, p=0.02)
- Global Assessment scores by study investigator increased (p<0.001) and the proportion of participants who improved was greater. (1+)

Table 7.8 Meta-analysis of COMT inhibitors compared with placebo[221] (1++)			
	Entacapone	**Tolcapone**	**Combined meta-analysis**
Number of trials	9	6	14
Sample size (N)	2,016	1,006	2,566
Efficacy			
Levodopa dose reduction	COMT[217,224–227,230]	COMT*[232–237]	COMT
Off time (hours)	COMT[217,224–227]	COMT*[232,233,235,236]	COMT
On time (hours)	COMT[217,224–227]	COMT*[232,233,235,236]	COMT
UPDRS ADL	COMT[217,225–227,231]	COMT**[234]	–
UPDRS motor score	COMT[217,225–227,231]	COMT**[233]	–
Adverse events			
Dyskinesia	P[224–227,231], NS[217]	P*[232–237]	P
Nausea	P[224–227,231], NS[217]	P*[232–237]	P
Vomiting	P[225,226], NS[217]	P*[232–237]	P
Diarrhoea	P[224–227], NS[217]	P**[233–235,237]	P
Constipation	P[224–226], NS[217]	NS[234–237]	
Hallucinations	NS[217,224–227]	P**[232–237]	P
Withdrawal rates			
Due to adverse events	P[224–227,231], NS[217]	NS[232–237]	P
Due to all causes	P[224–227,231], NS[217]	NS[232–237]	P

COMT = favouring COMT inhibitor (p<0.05); P = favouring placebo (p<0.05); – = not reported; NS = non-significant (p>0.05); *Significant for 50, 100, 200 and 400 mg tds doses; **Significant for 200 mg tds doses
Numbers within the table refer to the references of the original papers.

The RCT[222] also reported the following non-significant outcomes between treatment groups:

- Parkinson's Disease Questionnaire 39 (PDQ-39) summary index scores and subscores
- SF-36 variables and EQ-5D self-rating questionnaire utility score
- patient home diaries: mean 'off' time and mean 'on' time
- UPDRS I (mentation, behaviour and mood) scores
- dyskinesia sum score (UPDRS IVA)
- severity of PD (UPDRS part V; Hoehn and Yahr staging)
- UPDRS IV (Schwab and England)
- mean daily dose of levodopa. (1+)

The RCT[222] reported the following in relation to adverse events.

- 113 (65%) entacapone and 47 (49%) levodopa monotherapy people reported adverse events.
- A total of 311 adverse events occurred in entacapone (2.8 events per participant) and 104 in levodopa monotherapy group (2.2 events per participant).
- The most frequently reported adverse events significantly ($p<0.05$) in favour of levodopa monotherapy were nausea, diarrhoea, aggravated parkinsonism and constipation.
- A frequently reported adverse event was also dyskinesia, but there was no significant difference between treatment groups. (1+)

The RCT[222] reported the following results in relation to withdrawal rates.

- 45 (17%) of participants discontinued prematurely (27/174 entacapone and 18/96 levodopa monotherapy).
- Reported reasons for discontinuation were: adverse events for 26 (10%) of people; an unsatisfactory response to treatment for 14 (5%) of people; a wish to discontinue for three participants (1%); and other reasons for two participants (1%). (1+)

▷ From evidence to recommendation

The placebo-controlled COMT inhibitor trials document the efficacy of these agents in reducing off time and levodopa dose, while improving on time, motor impairments and disability. This is at the expense of increased dopaminergic adverse events such as nausea, vomiting and dyskinesia.

Tolcapone has caused rare cases of fatal hepatic toxicity and neuroleptic malignant syndrome. As a result, it can only be used in England and Wales after a patient has failed on entacapone and its use requires intensive monitoring of hepatic function (see Summary of Product Characteristics).

RECOMMENDATIONS

R44   Catechol-O-methyl transferase inhibitors may be used to reduce motor fluctuations in people with later PD.   **A**

R45   In view of problems with reduced concordance, people with later PD taking entacapone should be offered a triple combination preparation of levodopa, carbidopa and entacapone.*   **D (GPP)**

R46   Tolcapone should only be used after entacapone has failed in people with later PD due to lack of efficacy or side effects. Liver function tests are required every 2 weeks during the first year of therapy, and thereafter in accordance with the Summary of Product Characteristics.   **D (GPP)**

7.5.6 Amantadine

When originally introduced, amantadine was used as an early therapy for PD. It fell into disuse as more effective agents such as levodopa and dopamine agonists became available. In the last few years, amantadine has had a revival after several small trials suggested it might have an anti-dyskinetic effect in people with later PD and motor complications.

How effective and safe is amantadine in managing the motor complications of later PD?

---

*Trade name Stalevo® (Orion).

▷ Methodology

A Cochrane review[238] and an RCT[239] (published after the review) were found which compared the effectiveness of adding amantadine versus placebo in the treatment of people with later PD and motor complications.

The Cochrane review[238] included three studies with a total of 53 people, while the RCT[239] included a total of 40 people.

Issues for consideration included a lack of reporting: allocation concealment, washout periods in crossover design trials, clinical criteria for PD diagnosis, and intention-to-treat analysis. The trials were generally of small sample size (range 11–40) and short trial duration (range 4–6 weeks). A dose of 100–400 mg/day of amantadine was used.

The three trials[240–242] included in the review[238] were all crossover designs, in which none had reported the results of the first treatment arms. Two of the trials[241,242] did not incorporate a washout period; thus, data from these trials were not reported.

▷ Evidence statements

The RCT[239] found the results of key outcome measures changed over time (Table 7.9). (1+)

Table 7.9 Amantadine compared with placebo at different time points[239]			
	After 15 and 30 days' treatment	After 8 months' treatment	After 1 month withdrawal
Clinical rating scale			
UPDRS items 32–34 (self-assessment)	A	NS-B	NS
Motor complications			
IGA scores of dyskinesia	NS-A	NS-B	NS
DRS total scores	NS-A	NS-B	NS

A = favours amantadine (p<0.05); NS-A = non-significant improvement in amantadine; NS = no differences between groups; NS-B = non-significant worsening in amantadine; IGA = Investigator Global Assessment; DRS = Dyskinesia Rating Scale.

With respect to motor complications:
- Only one trial from the systematic review[240] reported the outcome of dyskinesia severity following levodopa challenge. This trial reported that dyskinesia was reduced after oral amantadine treatment by 6.4 points (41%) when compared with placebo arm (after 2 weeks of amantadine treatment). (1++)

With respect to adverse events:
- Only one trial[240] from the systematic review[238] reported adverse events for patients while on amantadine medication; these included: confusion, worsening of hallucinations, reappearance of palpitations, nausea, reversible oedema, dry mouth and constipation. (1++)

- Only one trial[239] from the review reported adverse events following amantadine withdrawal; these included: an abrupt increase of dyskinesia to 100% of daily time, hypothermia, and severe confusion (amantadine was reintroduced). (1+)

With respect to withdrawal rates:

- Reasons for withdrawal from amantadine treatment included: mild and transient adverse events,[242] tachycardia (N=1),[239] psychosis and livedo reticularis (N=2).[239] (1++)
- Reasons for withdrawal from placebo group included: dizziness,[239] somnolence,[239] poor compliance.[241] (1++)

▷ From evidence to recommendation

While there is some encouraging trial evidence that amantadine can be used as an anti-dyskinesia agent, data on its long-term effects are lacking. The evidence from one small trial suggests that amantadine's anti-dyskinetic effect is substantially reduced after 8 months of therapy. Further work is required in this area.

RECOMMENDATION

R47   Amantadine may be used to reduce dyskinesia in people with later PD.   C

7.5.7 Apomorphine

Apomorphine is a dopamine agonist that is not effective orally due to extensive first-pass metabolism in the liver. Early studies in PD lead to severe emesis and pre-renal failure. Its further development was facilitated by the availability of the antiemetic domperidone, which in doses of 10–30 mg tds for 72 hours before apomorphine can prevent most peripheral dopaminergic side effects.

There are currently two distinct methods of administering apomorphine: subcutaneous bolus doses and continuous infusion. People with a maximum of five or six off periods per day are suitable for intermittent bolus injections. Initially, the threshold dose of apomorphine (usual range 2–4 mg) is established as an inpatient using clinical examination and motor rating scales. The patient is then trained to use a pre-filled apomorphine injection system in which the agreed threshold dose can be dialled up more easily by the patient when in the off state.

Subcutaneous infusions of apomorphine are appropriate for PD people with so many off periods that repeated bolus injections are inappropriate. Apomorphine is administered by a portable syringe driver connected via a butterfly cannula sited in the abdominal wall or subcutaneous tissue of the thighs. The programmable pump delivers 50–120 mg of apomorphine over the waking day or the whole 24-hour period. Usually, oral medication can be reduced according to the patient's response. Considerable adjustment of the infusion dose is required once the patient is in the home environment. This can be facilitated by a PDNS.

What is the evidence that apomorphine injections and infusions are effective and safe treatments for motor complications in later PD?

7.5.8 Intermittent subcutaneous apomorphine injections

▷ Methodology

Three randomised controlled trials[243,244,245] were found which addressed the effectiveness of subcutaneous injections of apomorphine compared with placebo. The people included in these trials were all classified as later PD and had mean disease duration of 9–12 years.

All three studies[243,244,245] were placebo controlled. One was an 8-day crossover design[244] (4 days per arm), while another was a 4-week parallel design.[243] The third consisted of five N=1 trials conducted over 10 consecutive 'off periods' with each person acting as their own control[245]. The sample sizes of all three trials were relatively small (N=29,[243,244] N=22,[243,244] and N=5[245]).

No controlled trials were found which looked at apomorphine compared with standard oral treatment, and no controlled trials were found of continuous subcutaneous apomorphine infusions.

▷ Evidence statements

Table 7.10 summarises the evidence for subcutaneous apomorphine injections.

With respect to a correlation analysis:[243]
- Levodopa dose (the single dose that produced the effect to which apomorphine responses were matched) was not predictive of the required apomorphine dose.
- Total daily levodopa dose was also not predictive of apomorphine dose ($p=0.32$).
- Inpatient response was correlated with and predictive of outpatient efficacy ($p<0.001$). (1+)

With respect to clinical global impressions:[244]
- 86% of people who completed the apomorphine 8-week follow-up (maintenance phase) reported 'much' or 'very much' improvement at the last visit.
- No people reported to have worsened during the follow-up. (1+)

With respect to withdrawal rates:[243,244]
- Reasons for withdrawal included: failure to demonstrate a significant response to the levodopa challenge, adverse events (nausea and vomiting, hypotension, exanthema), lack of motivation. (1+)

With respect to adverse events:
- Common events included: injection site complaints, drowsiness, yawning, dyskinesias, nausea or vomiting, chorea, sweating and warmth, dizziness, headache, rhinitis.[243,244]
- Other events included: nausea, dyskinesia, short-lasting twinkling (sic) in legs, short-lasting worsening of tremor, warmth and sweating, lower level of motor functioning at end of clinical effect compared with basic level before the test.[245]
- There were no significant changes in other safety measures (blood tests, electrocardiography, physical examination).[243] (1+)

Table 7.10 Effectiveness of subcutaneous apomorphine injections (1+)

Outcome		Before versus after treatment
Clinical rating scales		
UPDRS (I, II, III, IV) scores		NS[244]
UPDRS motor (III) score		APO[243]
Columbia individual item (tremor, rigidity, gait, hypokinesia, stability) scores		APO[245]*
Columbia total score		APO[245]*
Timed finger/foot tapping, walking and pinboard combined test scores		APO[245]*
Patient diaries for hand-tapping test		APO[243]
Patient diaries for Webster step-seconds scores		p[243]
Motor complications		
Mean daily duration of off periods (minutes/day)	Staff rating	APO[244]
	Patient rating	APO[244]
Mean daily numbers of off periods	Staff rating	p[244]
	Patient rating	NS[244]
Distribution of severity of off periods		APO[244]
Patient diaries (out of 10 parameters):		
Off-state events aborted per patient		APO[243]
Onset latency (minutes)		APO[243]
Total time off per day		APO[243]
Incidence of dyskinesia		p[243]
Adverse events		
Yawning		p[243]
Mean daily duration of involuntary movements		p[243]
Mean daily numbers of involuntary movements		p[243]

APO = favouring dopamine agonist (p<0.05); *p <0.001; P = favouring placebo (p<0.05); – = not reported; NS = non-significant (p>0.05).

7.5.9 Apomorphine infusions

▷ Methodology

There were no randomised or controlled trials, which assessed the effectiveness of chronic apomorphine infusion in people with later PD. Ten studies, nine retrospective[246–254] and one prospective,[255] were found which investigated the benefit of chronic apomorphine treatment compared with pre-treatment evaluations.

Most of the included retrospective studies used a hospital/clinic database to identify people who had received apomorphine for the treatment of severe motor fluctuations or dyskinesia, but who were refractory to optimal oral medication. One prospective study enrolled people with motor fluctuations and dyskinesias at two sites if they were refractory to oral medication and scheduled to start continuous apomorphine infusion.[255] For included studies, the follow-up ranged from 3 months to 5 years, the sample size ranged from seven to 64 people, and the average age ranged from 56 to 65 years.

The methodological limitations of these studies included: lack of prospective protocols in most instances, non-randomisation of people, lack of control groups, small sample sizes, and lack of patient and/or investigator blinding.

▷ Evidence statements

Table 7.11 summarises the evidence for continuous apomorphine infusions.

With respect to clinical global rating scales:[250]
- Patient rating: no patient described overall worsening; three felt unchanged; six experienced slight improvement; and 16 had a clear improvement.[250]
- Physician rating: no patient worsened; two people were unchanged (the same who described themselves as unchanged); seven slightly improved; and 16 had clearly improved. (3)

With respect to drug dosage:[252]
- Larger doses of apomorphine produced a longer duration of anti-parkinsonian effect ($p<0.001$). (3)
- Two studies[253,254] looked at the anti-dyskinetic effect of monotherapy, which means these people received no oral anti-parkinsonian drug treatment from the time when the apomorphine pump was started in the morning to when it was turned off at night. There was an overlap in the patient populations included in these studies; therefore, only the results of one [253] will be reported below.

With respect to motor complications:[253]
- There was a mean maximum reduction of dyskinesia per patient of 64% ($p<0.005$).
- The mean time to achieve maximum dyskinesia improvement was 12.1 months.
- There was an increase in on time of 55% ($p<0.005$). (3)

With respect to treatment management:[253]
- 25% of people managed treatment independently, 50% managed with family help, 25% required nurse input.
- The success rate was greater ($p<0.05$, 81%) among people managing the pump system independently or with help from family than those requiring outside help (eg nurse). (3)

Table 7.11 Effectiveness of continuous apomorphine infusions (3)	
Outcome	**Before versus after treatment**
Clinical rating scales	
UPDRS total and subscores	APO[247]
UPDRS 32 (dyskinesia duration)	APO[255]*
UPDRS 33 (dyskinesia severity)	APO[255]
Lang and Fahn	APO[255]
Hoehn and Yahr scores (off and on states)	APO[250]
Schwab and England scale (off and on states)	APO[250]
Severity and duration in diaries	APO[255]*
Motor complications	
Decrease in off time	APO[246–248,250–253, 255]
Increase in on-time duration (% waking day)	APO[255]*
Dyskinesias	NS[247,248,250]
Levodopa	
Daily dose of levodopa	APO[246–250,252,255]*
Number of levodopa doses per day	APO[252]

APO = favouring apomorphine treatment (p<0.05); *p<0.01; NS = non-significant.

With respect to neuropsychiatric problems:[253]

- There was 40% improvement (especially in people with depressive-type symptoms) (p<0.05). **(3)**

With respect to adverse events:[246–253,255]

- The majority of people developed subcutaneous nodules.
- Other effects were: rhinorrhoea, nausea and hiccups, recurrent diarrhoea, confusion and emotional lability, euphoria and dysarthria, worsening of dyskinesia, orthostatic hypotension, psychosis, hallucinations, intermittent illusions, confusion, sleepiness, vertigo, eosinophilia, increased appetite, increased libido, visual delusions, diurnal agitation, immune haemolytic anaemia, mild self-limiting leg oedema, positive direct anti-globulin test without associated haematological changes. **(3)**

With respect to withdrawal rates:[246,248,250–253]

- People withdrew due to side effects (psychiatric effects, insufficient therapeutic effects or adverse effects). **(3)**

With respect to effects of single-dose levodopa and apomorphine challenges before and after continuous apomorphine infusion on dyskinesias:[255]

- Levodopa reduced dyskinesias after continuous apomorphine infusion by at least 40% (AIMS and Goetz scales; both p<0.01).
- Apomorphine reduced dyskinesias after continuous apomorphine infusion by at least 36% (AIMS and Goetz scales; both p<0.01). (3)

▷ From evidence to recommendation

The evidence base for the use of both intermittent injections and continuous infusions of apomorphine is relatively poor but both techniques are licensed for use in England and Wales. The GDG considers these to be useful treatment modalities for people with severe off periods that are not responsive to changes in oral medication. However, there is a risk of triggering serious side effects such as confusion and hallucinations. In addition, the risk of injection site reactions is considerable.

Long-term continuous apomorphine infusions can dramatically reduce both off periods and dyskinesia and allow withdrawal of oral medication.

The initiation of apomorphine should be restricted to expert units with the availability of a home monitoring system by a suitably trained health professional such as a PDNS.

RECOMMENDATIONS

R48   Intermittent apomorphine injections may be used to reduce off time in people with PD with severe motor complications.   **B**

R49   Continuous subcutaneous infusions of apomorphine may be used to reduce off time and dyskinesia in people with PD with severe motor complications. Its initiation should be restricted to expert units with facilities for appropriate monitoring.   **D**

7.6   Comparisons of drug classes

While it is valuable to know that various drug classes are effective agents in managing the motor complications seen in later PD, clinicians are particularly keen to know whether one class or combination of classes is better than another so that clinicians can make rational decisions about the order in which adjuvant therapies are used.

7.6.1   Dopamine agonists compared with monoamine oxidase type B inhibitors

How effective are dopamine agonists compared with MAOB inhibitors in the management of later PD?

▷ Methodology

No trials were found which compared dopamine agonists with MAOB inhibitors in the treatment of people with later PD and motor complications.

▷ From evidence to recommendation

In the absence of any evidence, no firm conclusions on the comparative efficacy and safety of dopamine agonists versus MAOB inhibitors can be made. Further trials are required to compare these two drug classes.

7.6.2 Catechol-O-methyl transferase inhibitors compared with dopamine agonists

How effective are dopamine agonists compared with COMT inhibitors in the management of later PD?

▷ Methodology

One Cochrane review[256] was found which compared the effectiveness of dopamine agonists versus COMT inhibitors.

Two RCTs were included in the review. One trial[257] (N=205) compared tolcapone with pergolide and the other trial[258] (N=146) compared tolcapone with bromocriptine.

▷ Evidence statements

With respect to quality of life:[257]
- PDQ-39 improved more with tolcapone than pergolide (p=0.005).
- Sickness Impact Profile was non-significant. (1++)

With respect to clinical rating scales:[257,258]
- Both studies found a non-significant difference in UPDRS ADL scores and UPDRS motor scores. (1++)

With respect to levodopa dose reduction:
- One trial[258] found the total daily levodopa dose decreased significantly with tolcapone compared with bromocriptine (124 mg versus 30 mg, p<0.01).
- The other trial[257] found a non-significant difference between tolcapone and pergolide (mean of 108 mg versus 92 mg). (1++)

With respect to total on and off time:
- One trial[258] found a non-significant difference in off and on time between tolcapone and bromocriptine. (1++)

With respect to adverse events:
- The combined results of both trials showed more nausea (OR=0.42, p=0.0003), constipation (OR=0.26, p=0.00007) and orthostatic complaints (OR=0.24, p=0.0002) in pergolide and bromocriptine groups than in tolcapone groups. (1++)

With respect to withdrawal rates:
- One of the studies[257] reported, due to adverse events, a trend towards more pergolide withdrawals (Peto OR=0.34, p=0.02). Neither study showed any significant differences for all-cause withdrawal. (1++)

▷ From evidence to recommendation

While there is some evidence of the superiority of tolcapone over bromocriptine and pergolide, this is insufficient to recommend the use of COMT inhibitors ahead of dopamine agonists. Further trials are required to compare these classes of adjuvant therapy.

7.6.3 Dopamine agonists compared with amantadine

How effective are dopamine agonists compared with amantadine in the management of later PD?

▷ Methodology

No trials were found which compared adding dopamine agonists versus amantadine to levodopa therapy in the treatment of people with later PD and motor complications.

▷ From evidence to recommendation

In the absence of any evidence, no conclusions on the comparative efficacy and safety of dopamine agonists compared with amantadine can be made. Further trials are required to compare these two drug classes.

7.7 Choice of pharmacological therapy in later Parkinson's disease

7.7.1 From evidence to recommendation

A summary of the drugs covered in this section can be found in Table 7.4.

It was evident from reviewing the evidence base that there is no single drug of choice in the pharmacotherapy of later PD.

Further trials are required in later PD with motor fluctuations to compare adjuvant therapy with dopamine agonists, COMT inhibitors and MAOB inhibitors, preferably using quality-of-life and health economics outcome measures. The PD MED trial in the UK is just such a trial and is scheduled to continue recruitment until November 2006 (**www.pdmed.bham.ac.uk**).

7.7.2 Generic therapeutic issues in later Parkinson's disease

There are a number of generic issues concerning the prescription and administration of anti-parkinsonian medication that are crucial to good concordance. Sudden increases in off time can occur if people with later PD are not given their medication often enough when they are admitted to hospital or care homes. This may require administration at times other than the normal 'drug rounds'. This is often best achieved by allowing patients to self-medicate. It is also advisable that the anti-parkinsonian regimen of patients admitted to hospital is reviewed and, if necessary, adjusted by an expert.

In addition, there are concerns over the dangers of sudden withdrawal or changes in medication and the overuse of such medication by a minority of people with PD.

RECOMMENDATIONS

R50   It is not possible to identify a universal first-choice adjuvant drug therapy for people with later PD. The choice of adjuvant drug first prescribed should take into account:

- clinical and lifestyle characteristics
- patient preference, after the patient has been informed of the short- and long-term benefits and drawbacks of the drug classes.   **D (GPP)**

R51   Anti-parkinsonian medication should not be withdrawn abruptly or allowed to fail suddenly due to poor absorption (for example gastroenteritis, abdominal surgery) to avoid the potential for acute akinesia or neuroleptic malignant syndrome.   **D (GPP)**

R52   The practice of withdrawing patients from their anti-parkinsonian drugs (so-called 'drug holidays') to reduce motor complications should not be undertaken because of the risk of neuroleptic malignant syndrome.   **D (GPP)**

R53   In view of the risks of sudden changes in anti-parkinsonian medication, people with PD who are admitted to hospital or care homes should have their medication:

- given at the appropriate times, which in some cases may mean allowing self-medication
- adjusted by, or adjusted only after discussion with, a specialist in the management of PD.   **D (GPP)**

R54   Clinicians should be aware of dopamine dysregulation syndrome, an uncommon disorder in which dopaminergic medication misuse is associated with abnormal behaviours, including hypersexuality, pathological gambling and stereotypic motor acts. This syndrome may be difficult to manage.   **D (GPP)**

8 | Surgery for Parkinson's disease

8.1 | Introduction

Recognition of the limitations of dopaminergic therapy and the need to treat motor complications were the prime movers in the revival of functional stereotactic surgery for PD. This was aided by technological advances in the fields of imaging and computing. The introduction of CT and MRI scanning allowed surgeons to visualise and directly target deep brain structures without the need for indirect calculations from atlases based on cadaveric dissections. Modern engineering methods and computer technology resulted in easily used and reliable stereotactic hardware. Further advances came with the development of technology for deep brain stimulation (DBS), which has become the mainstay of movement disorder surgery.

Better understanding of the pathophysiology of movement disorders and of the basal ganglia circuitry has refined the surgical targets used in movement disorder surgery.

The ventrolateral nucleus of the thalamus has been one of the commonly used target sites for surgery in PD. Cells firing at tremor frequency can be identified in the ventralis intermedius (Vim) part of the thalamus and lesions or stimulators placed at this target can dramatically improve tremor.[259]

The serendipitous observation[260] of the effects of accidental ligation of the anterior choroidal artery focused attention on the globus pallidus interna (GPi) as a target for surgery. One group[261] identified the ventral and posterior parts of the internal segment (GPi) as the optimal site for surgical ablation. This group[261] revived this procedure and it was in widespread use in the early 1990s. While pallidotomy significantly reduced dyskinesia, it had a lesser effect on tremor and akinesia. The morbidity of bilateral lesions and the introduction of subthalamic nucleus (STN) DBS reduced the use of pallidotomy. However, DBS of the pallidum has a role in dystonia and some patients with PD.

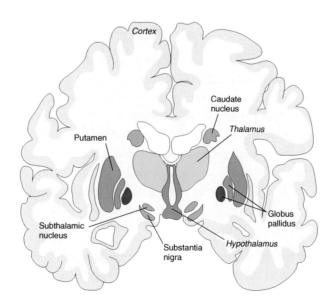

Figure 8.1 Structures of the basal ganglia[262] (reproduced with permission from publisher).

Experimental studies using the MPTP primate model showed increased cellular activity in the STN, and lesions or stimulation of the STN can reverse the cardinal features of parkinsonism.[263,264] However, surgeons were reluctant to lesion the STN in humans because of the risk of inducing hemiballismus. It was then shown that electrical stimulation of the STN-DBS[265] produced dramatic improvement in parkinsonian symptoms in PD. STN-DBS has since become the most widely undertaken surgical procedure for PD.

Surgical techniques vary between centres, but it is generally performed in three stages: radiological localisation, physiological localisation, and then either an ablation or a stimulation procedure.

Radiological localisation involves the rigid fixation to the skull under local anaesthesia of a stereotactic base ring onto which a fiducial array can be mounted. In the past, ventriculography (ie outlining the ventricles of the brain by instilling air or contrast medium) was the radiological technique used, but this has been largely replaced by CT and MRI. It is now possible to identify most of the targets on MRI, and their position in stereotactic space is calculated using sophisticated computer programs.

When the radiological data have been acquired and analysed, the patient is moved to the operating theatre and the radiological localiser is replaced with a stereotactic arc system that allows the surgeon to pass electrodes through a small opening in the skull with a high degree of precision. This is usually undertaken under local anaesthesia to allow the surgeon to evaluate responses from the patient, though some centres now carry this out under general anaesthesia and depend on recording of cellular activity for final localisation of the target. Microelectrode recording of cellular activity is widely used for physiological localisation, but there is no consensus on the added value of this technique. Evaluating the patient's response to electrical stimulation of the target usually makes further confirmation of accurate identification of the target.

When the target has been identified the options are of either using radiofrequency current for thermal ablation of the area or introducing a system for chronic electrical stimulation. Ablation has the advantage of being an inexpensive single procedure that does not require long-term follow-up for maintenance of implanted hardware. These advantages are largely negated by the irreversibility of the procedure and higher morbidity. Ablation has therefore largely been replaced by chronic DBS.

For DBS, the initial target localization is similar to that used for ablative procedures. Once the target has been identified the test electrode is replaced with an implantable quadripolar electrode, which is anchored to the skull. A period of stimulation using an external stimulator is sometimes used and when the efficacy has been confirmed the system is internalised. Under general anaesthesia fine cables are connected to the electrodes and tunnelled subcutaneously to a programmable pulse generator usually placed in the chest wall. The pulse generator is similar to a cardiac pacemaker with a high degree of programmability by an external device. It is possible to provide the patient with a degree of control of the stimulator. The pulse generator has a battery within it and depending on usage will have to be replaced in a simple surgical procedure every 3–5 years.

In view of the relative safety of stimulation procedures compared with lesioning, most surgery for people with PD today uses the former approach. The GDG felt therefore that it should confine its recommendations to STN, GPi and thalamic stimulation.

8.1.1 Methodological limitations of surgery trials

The included trials all had methodological limitations common to non-analytical study designs. Firstly, none of the included trials were randomised into surgical or non-surgical intervention groups. Secondly, none of the trials were performed under blinded conditions, either single or double. None of the trials were controlled with a cohort of non-surgical patients for longitudinal comparison over time.

There was also a general lack of inclusion/exclusion criteria, which could lead to pre-selected patient populations, lack of multi-centre comparative results analysis, and lack of sample size calculations. The mean follow-up of most trials was 7–12 months and the patient population tended to be younger with an average age of approximately 60 years.

What is the effectiveness and safety of any DBS procedure versus standard medical therapy in the treatment of motor complications in patients with PD?

8.2 Subthalamic nucleus stimulation

8.2.1 Methodology

No randomised or controlled trials were found on the effectiveness of any DBS procedure versus standard medical therapy. Therefore, the GDG agreed that large case series studies with a minimum sample size of 40 patients were to be accepted for review.

Nine papers were found which reported the effectiveness of STN-DBS versus standard medical therapy.

8.2.2 Health economic methodology

Four health economic studies met our quality criteria.[266-269] One study[267] evaluated the incremental cost-effectiveness of bilateral DBS of the STN or GPi versus best medical management. The study[267] estimated the cost per QALY of bilateral DBS of the STN or GPi (intervention) versus best medical management in the US healthcare context.

Another study[266] evaluated the incremental cost-effectiveness of STN-DBS versus drug treatment. This study[266] estimated the extra cost per additional UPDRS point gained from bilateral high-frequency STN-DBS by comparing STN-DBS and drug treatment with drug treatment alone in the German healthcare context.

One study[268] evaluated the costs of STN-DBS. The study[268] estimated the total health service cost per patient including preoperative assessment, STN-DBS and postoperative management over a 5-year period in the UK healthcare context.

Another study[269] evaluated the change in medication costs after bilateral STN-DBS. This study[269] estimated the anti-parkinsonian medication costs pre- and post-operatively at 1 and 2 years after bilateral STN-DBS in a US healthcare context.

A simplified cost-effectiveness analysis of bilateral DBS-STN was estimated from the perspective of the NHS over 5-year period (Appendix F).

8.2.3 Evidence statements

With respect to quality of life:[270]

- Parkinsonian symptoms, systemic symptoms, emotional functioning and social functioning all improved post-operatively (p<0.001).
- The improvement in the score of UPDRS II correlated with the improvement in total Parkinson's Disease Quality of Life (PDQL) score (p<0.001). (3)

With respect to efficacy, see Table 8.1.

Table 8.1 Bilateral STN stimulation (stimulator 'on')						
	3 months	6 months	1 year	2 years	3 years	5 years
Quality of life						
PDQL	–	–	S[270]	–	–	–
Clinical rating scales						
Hoehn and Yahr	–	S[271,272]	S[272]	S[272]	–	–
UPDRS I∫	–	–	NS[270]	–	B[273]	–
UPDRS II∫	S[273,274]	S[271,272]	S[270,272–274] NS[275] B*[275]	S[272,274]	–	S[276]
UPDRS III	S[273,274]	S[271]	S[270,273–275]	S[274]	–	S[276]
UPDRS IV	S[274]	S[271]	S[274]	S[274]	–	–
SEALD∫	S[273]	S[272]	S[270,272,273,276]	S[272]	S[276]	S[276]
BDI	–	–	S[270,273]	–	S[273]	NS[276]
Motor complications						
Tremor	S[273]	S[272]	S[272,273]	S[272]	–	S[276]
Dyskinesias (on drug)	–	S[272]	S[270,272,275] NS[273]	S[272]	–	–
Dystonia ∫	–	S[272]	S[272] NS[273]	S[272]	–	–
Akinesia and rigidity	S[273]	S[272]	S[272,273]	S[272]	–	S[276]
Axial symptoms^	–	S[271,272]	S[271,272]	S[272]	–	–
Fluctuations	–	S[271]	S[275]	–	–	–
Medication						
Levodopa dose	S[274]	S[271,272]	S[270,272,274–276] NS[273]	S[272,274]	S[276]	S[276]

S = improvement in favour of STN stimulation (p<0.05); NS = not-significant; B = worsening of symptoms after surgery (p<0.05); – = not reported; * = patients >70 years of age; ^ = axial symptoms: speech, postural stability and gait (items 18, 28, 29 and 30 of UPDRS III); ∫ = off medication.

With respect to predictive factors, the following results were observed (Table 8.2):

- One study[274] found: 'the younger the age at the moment of operation and the shorter the duration of disease, the better the clinical outcome'. Another study[271] reported: no significant correlation between age at time of surgery or disease duration and post-operative clinical outcome. (3)
- One study[275] found: UPDRS motor scores off medication were improved but less so in patients over 70 (<70 vs >70, p<0.02), and changes in UPDRS motor scores (on medication) worsened in patients over 70 and improved in patients under 70 (p<0.05). Another study[274] found: no significant difference between patients older and younger than 60 years of age for UPDRS II, III and IV scores, and no significant difference in mean daily levodopa dosage at follow-up. (3)

Table 8.2 Correlations between pre-operative and post-operative factors

Pre-operative factor	Correlation	Post-operative outcome
Age[275]	–	Improvement from stimulation (p<0.01)
Age of patients[273]	–	Frontal score (p<0.001) and initiation subset of Mattis DRS (p=0.007)
Age of patients[273]	–	Item 2 of UPDRS thought disorders (p=0.023)
Age or disease duration (p<0.005 and p<0.007 respectively)[271]	+	Motor disability score in the 'on' stimulation and 'on' drug conditions
Younger patients and shorter disease duration[271]	+	Residual ADL, motor disability and axial scores
Low motor disability and high neuropsychological status[271]	+	Improvement in motor disability *Please note: low motor disability predicting level of improvement in motor disability after surgery may be a statistical artefact (regression to mean).*
Less severe axial motor symptoms[271]	+	Improvement in axial motor disability
Levodopa challenge[275]	+	Results from STN-DBS (p<0.02)
Improvement from levodopa[275]	+	Improvement from STN-DBS (p<0.00001)
Levodopa response in an individual symptom[275]	+	Stimulation response for that same symptom (akinesia, tremor, rigidity, postural instability, gait and pull test (p<0.001))
Improvement from levodopa in Hoehn and Yahr and Schwab and England global ratings[275]	+	Improvement from stimulation in the same rating (p<0.001)

+ = Positively correlated (ie increase in factor 1 leads to an increase in factor 2); − = negatively correlated (ie increase in factor 1 leads to a decrease in factor 2)

With respect to adverse events, the following were reported following STN-DBS:

- Neuropsychological events including: confusion, mania, delusion, depression, hypomania, aggressive behaviour, hallucinations, attentional and cognitive deficit, dementia, panic attack and apathy, which in some impaired activities of daily living.
- Other adverse events including: hypophonia, transitory eye opening apraxia, thrombophlebitis, subcutaneous infection, haematomas, focal cerebral contusions, infections of the system (sic) ('the system' relates to the actual equipment used), dysarthria, disequilibrium, dystonia, weight gain, connection wound dehiscence, lead repositioning, air embolus, seizure and dyskinesias.
- Stimulator-induced events including: electrode replacement due to unsatisfactory results, local pain at the implantation site of the pulse generator, reversible stimulation-induced dyskinesias after an increase in voltage, minor intracerebral bleeding at the site of the trajectory lead, dislocation of the impulse generator from site of implantation, transient paraesthesias associated with adjustment of stimulation parameter. (3)

With respect to withdrawal rates:

- Two studies reported suicide attempts: one study reported patients with depression (three) who then attempted suicide (two)[270] and the other study reported four patients who attempted suicide post-operatively (one died).[273]
- In a third study,[277] three patients died from causes unrelated to surgery or stimulation, and in a fourth study[276] three deaths were reported (from intracerebral haemorrhage, myocardial infarction and suicide). (3)

8.2.4 Health economic evidence statements

Bilateral STN- or GPi-DBS costs an additional \$49,194 in US\$2000 (approximately £31,112) per QALY in comparison to best medical management.[267] The study's results suggest DBS may therefore be cost-effective if the quality of life after the procedure is improved by 18% or more compared with best medical management.

Bilateral STN-DBS costs approximately an additional DM1,800 (UK£580) in 2002 prices per unit improvement in UPDRS total score, derived from German costs and patient data.[266] However, the costs will decrease further over the long term (> 1 year study period) from reduced drug expenditure and improved patient functioning. Therefore, the direct and indirect costs need to be assessed over the long term to sufficiently evaluate the cost-effectiveness of DBS.

The total health service costs of DBS of the STN, including pre-operative assessment, surgery and post-operative management over a 5-year period, was recently evaluated in the UK.[268] The estimated total cost per patient was £32,526 for the bilateral procedure and £30,447 for the unilateral procedure (£ 2002).[268]

A US study evaluated the change in anti-parkinsonian medication costs 2 years after bilateral STN-DBS. The study found the medication costs had significantly decreased by 32% ($p \leq 0.01$) from the 1-year pre-operative costs and there was 39% reduction after 2 years.[269] Pre-operatively, the average daily cost of PD medication was \$19.53 ± 10.41 in US\$ 2002 (approximately £11.92 ± 6.35) per patient. Post-operatively, this fell to \$13.25 ± 5.41 (approximately £8.08 ± 3.30) per patient.[269]

The economic modelling performed for this guideline (Appendix F) suggests that STN-DBS costs approximately £19,500 per QALY over a 5-year period in comparison to standard PD care in the UK (£ 1998). The results are relatively robust based on one-way sensitivity analysis.

8.2.5 From evidence to recommendation

In the absence of RCTs, any conclusions on the efficacy and safety of bilateral STN stimulation must be tentative. Most of the patients in the open-label non-controlled trials described above were relatively young (aged around 60 years) so the results may not be generalisable to all those with the condition. Follow-up was for around 12 months only, which may not record later complications.

Despite these limitations, what evidence is available supports the efficacy of this technique in reducing off time, dyskinesia and levodopa dose, improving motor impairments and disability, and improving quality of life.

There is a small but significant risk of permanent neurological disability as a consequence of this operation, due mostly to cerebral infarction or haemorrhage. In a small number of patients, this can lead to death. Most other adverse effects of surgery were transient but concern remains regarding the incidence of neuropsychiatric complications, particularly depression and suicide. It is difficult to comment reliably on such issues in the absence of a control group.

The procedure requires an experienced, well-trained multidisciplinary team.

The high cost of this type of functional neurosurgery in PD is well recognised. No long-term data from clinical trials are available. However, economic modelling over a 5-year period performed as part of this guideline suggests that bilateral STN-DBS costs £19,500 per QALY in comparison to standard PD care in the UK (£ 1998).

The National Institute for Health and Clinical Excellence (NICE) published an Interventional Procedure Statement on bilateral STN stimulation in November 2003.[23] This supported the use of the procedure provided normal arrangements for consent, audit and clinical governance are in place.

The PD SURG trial is evaluating the clinical and cost-effectiveness of STN surgery and recruitment is ongoing (**www.pdsurg.bham.ac.uk/**). The NICE Interventional Procedure Statement encouraged clinicians to consider randomising patients in this trial.

RECOMMENDATION

R55   Bilateral STN stimulation may be used in people with PD who:
- have motor complications that are refractory to best medical treatment,
- are biologically fit with no clinically significant active comorbidity,
- are levodopa responsive and
- have no clinically significant active mental health problems, for example depression or dementia.   **D**

8.3   Globus pallidus interna stimulation

8.3.1   Methodology

No randomised or controlled trials were found on the effectiveness of any GPi-DBS procedure versus standard medical therapy. Therefore, large case series designs with a minimum sample size of 40 people were accepted for review.

8.3.2   Evidence statements

No trials were found which assessed the effectiveness of GPi stimulation in a case series with a minimum sample size of 40 people with PD.

8.3.3   From evidence to recommendation

While no RCTs or large case series have evaluated GPi-DBS, there are a small number of case series and comparative trials that suggest the procedure is effective (see section 8.4). However, it is likely to suffer from the same concerns regarding adverse events and costs as STN-DBS.

GPi-DBS is rarely performed for PD in the UK at present, though it is sometimes undertaken when STN-DBS is not possible.

RECOMMENDATION

R56   Bilateral GPi stimulation may be used in people with PD who:
- have motor complications that are refractory to best medical treatment,
- are biologically fit with no clinically significant active comorbidity,
- are levodopa responsive and
- have no clinically significant active mental health problems, for example depression or dementia.   D (GPP)

8.4   Comparison of different types of deep brain stimulation

What is the most effective form of DBS procedure in the treatment of motor fluctuations and complications in patients with PD?

8.4.1   Methodology

There were no randomised or controlled trials reporting the most effective form of DBS in the treatment of patients with PD. The majority of trials were retrospective case series, which compared the results of different techniques. Due to the lack of comparative trials in this area, the GDG agreed studies with a sample size minimum of 10 patients per arm should be reviewed.

Five trials[278–282] were found which compared the before and after surgery results of STN-, GPi- and Vim thalamic DBS.

The majority of the patient population received bilateral implantation, though results were not reported separately from the unilateral implantation results.

8.4.2 Evidence statements

With respect to clinical efficacy

- The following criteria were significantly (p<0.05) in favour of both STN- and GPi-DBS:
  - UPDRS I, II (off and on), III (off and on), IV[278,279,281,282]
  - time in off state (UPDRS item 39)[282]
  - Hoehn and Yahr scores[281]
  - levodopa equivalent daily dose[278,279,281]
  - dyskinesia scores[278,279]
  - patient and physician global assessments
  - Schwab and England scale[282]
  - home diary scores (% of time with good mobility and without dyskinesia during the waking day).[279] (3)
- The following criteria were improved in only one DBS technique versus another:
  - Motor score improvement was more pronounced in STN patients than GPi patients (no p values stated).[281]
  - Medication could be reduced only in STN patients and not in GPi patients (no p values stated).[281]
  - Levodopa dose equivalent, though unchanged in the GPi group, was significantly reduced in the STN group (p=0.017).[282]
  - Trail making test (p=0.0013), test B (p=0.0015) and BDI (p<0.0001) improved under STN stimulation and not Gpi.[281]
  - Literal (p=0.0018) and total (p=0.0002) fluency decreased under STN-DBS and not GPi-DBS.[281]
  - Core Assessment Program for Intracerebral Transplantations dyskinesia rating scale favoured GPi (p=0.046) in absolute scores but percentage changes were not significant.[282] (3)
- Thalamic nucleus stimulation could not be compared directly to other techniques, as the outcome measures used to assess its efficacy are different from other techniques. The main outcome, tremor suppression, was found to be significantly improved with the procedure.[283] (3)

With respect to adverse events, the following was reported:

- No GPi-specific adverse events were reported.
- See thalamic stimulation and STN stimulation sections for events specific to these procedures. (3)

8.4.3 From evidence to recommendation

There is no evidence from RCTs to compare STN with GPi stimulation. However, observational studies suggest that STN stimulation may lead to greater improvement in motor scores and more reduction in levodopa dose and depression scores. In comparison, GPi stimulation may lead to less cognitive impairment. Further work is required in this area.

It is recognised that pallidal stimulation for PD is rarely performed at present, though it is sometimes undertaken when STN-DBS is not possible.

RECOMMENDATION

R57   With the current evidence it is not possible to decide if the STN or GPi is the preferred target for DBS for people with PD, or whether one form of surgery is more effective or safer than the other. In considering the type of surgery, account should be taken of:

- clinical and lifestyle characteristics of the person with PD
- patient preference after the patient has been informed of the potential benefits and drawbacks of the different surgical procedures.   **D (GPP)**

8.5   Thalamic stimulation

How effective and safe is thalamic stimulation for the control of tremor in PD?

8.5.1   Methodology

Three papers[284,283,285] reported the effectiveness of chronic stimulation to the Vim thalamic nuclei. The methodological limitations of these papers are similar to those of STN stimulation (see Section 8.2).

8.5.2   Evidence statements

With respect to tremor suppression:

- All three studies[284,283,285] showed a benefit of thalamic stimulation.
- Only one study[283] reported statistical analysis and stated that the following outcomes were significantly ($p<0.05$) improved: face tremor and observed tremor, hypokinesia, rigidity and ADL score. **(3)**

With respect to adverse events, the following were reported:

- Post-operative events included: venous infarction with temporary aphasia, intraventricular haemorrhage and cardiovascular problems intra-operatively.
- Stimulation-related events that occurred considerably more frequently in patients with bilateral implants (52%) as compared with unilateral (31%)[285] included: dystonia, diplopia, sleepiness, altered mental status, paraesthesias, mild disturbance of gait and balance, mild dysarthria, increased drooling, nausea, insomnia, dysphagia, depression, wire tightness and dysarthria. **(3)**
- No mortality was reported in any of the trials.

With respect to withdrawal rates:

- Most withdrawals were due to adverse events. **(3)**

8.5.3 From evidence to recommendation

There is no evidence from RCTs of the benefit of thalamic stimulation in PD. Data from observational studies suggest that this is an effective method of reducing tremor. The operation carries a risk of serious complications such as cerebral infarction and haemorrhage. The GDG recognised that this form of surgery is rarely performed for tremor in people with PD in England and Wales, having been superseded by STN stimulation.

RECOMMENDATION

R58   Thalamic DBS may be considered as an option in people with PD who predominantly have severe disabling tremor and where STN stimulation cannot be performed.   **D**

9 Non-motor features of Parkinson's disease

'I feel trapped inside my body . . . as if I'm not in control . . . almost as if someone or something else is running my life.' (patient)[2]

9.1 Introduction

The spectrum of PD includes many problems that do not directly affect motor function. These non-motor features are of crucial importance to people since they have a major impact on quality of life.[28,286]

Non-motor features comprise:
- mental health problems
- depression and dementia
- falls and potential fractures
- sleep disturbance
- autonomic disturbance and pain.

While most people are troubled by these problems in the later stages of their PD, certain non-motor conditions can develop throughout the course of the condition (eg depression, anxiety, hypersomnolence) or even precede it (eg sleep disturbance, depression, anxiety).

A recent study reported on the non-motor problems experienced by a group of 149 people with PD followed for 15–18 years.[287] They found the occurrence rates were: falls 81% (with 23% suffering fractures), cognitive decline 84% (48% fulfilling criteria for dementia), hallucinations 50%, depression 50%, choking 50%, symptomatic postural hypotension 35%, and urinary incontinence 41%.

There have previously been few therapeutic studies examining the effects of treatments for non-motor disorders. However, there is now a real desire to increase research into the non-motor features of PD as their effect on people's well-being has been recognised.[288]

The non-motor features of PD considered in the scope of this guideline and thus undergoing literature review were:
- mental health problems:
  - depression
  - dementia
  - psychosis
- sleep disturbance:
  - hypersomnolence
  - rapid eye movement sleep behaviour disorder (RBD)
  - restless legs syndrome (RLS)
  - inverted sleep-wake cycle
  - nocturnal akinesia.

Although the following non-motor features of PD were not considered within the scope of this guideline, it is recognised that they are important and should always be considered in patient care. These non-motor features include:

- mental health problems
  - anxiety
  - apathy
- falls
- autonomic disturbance
  - bowel dysfunction including constipation
  - dysphagia
  - weight loss
  - dribbling of saliva
  - bladder dysfunction
  - sexual dysfunction
  - postural hypotension
  - excessive sweating
- pain.

Depression, dementia and psychosis are frequent problems in PD and some research has been performed on their treatment. Therefore, these topics were included in the scope of this guideline.

Other important mental health issues in PD include anxiety and apathy, but little work has been done in these areas specific to PD so they were not included in the scope. Standard treatment therefore applies in these areas; see NICE guidance entitled: 'Anxiety: management of anxiety (panic disorder, with or without agoraphobia, and generalised anxiety disorder) in adults in primary, secondary and community care'.[21]

9.2 Mental health problems

9.2.1 Depression

Depression affects around 40–50% of people with PD.[289] It is usually mild to moderate but can be severe, and symptoms of depression can predate motor manifestations.

The relationship of depression to the pathology of PD is unclear but the inconsistent relationship between mood changes and the severity of motor symptoms indicates that depression should not simply be considered a reaction to motor disability.

There are difficulties in diagnosing mild depression in people with PD as the clinical features of depression overlap with the motor features of PD.

The characteristic features of depression are low mood, loss of interest and enjoyment, and fatigue. This is accompanied by various combinations of:

- slowed mental and physical function
- motor agitation
- poor appetite and sleep
- weight loss

- other somatic symptoms
- disturbance of cognitive function and thought processes.

The disturbance of cognitive functions and thought processes may result in poor concentration and memory, excessive worry, feelings of worthlessness, hopelessness and guilt, negative views of self and life, and thoughts of suicide. Psychological and physical symptoms of anxiety are also common.

The development of depression creates an added burden for people with PD and their carers and has been shown to be an important determinant of quality of life.[290]

Factors relevant to the aetiology of depression that need to be considered are:
- previous susceptibility to depression
- neurotransmitter disturbances of PD
- effects of drug treatments
- relationship to on–off motor fluctuations
- the person's adjustment to the diagnosis of PD and their symptoms and life factors, including losses
- other stressors
- interpersonal relationships.

What is the effectiveness of antidepressant therapies versus placebo or active comparator in the treatment of depression in PD?

▷ Methodology

A Cochrane review[291] and two randomised controlled trials[292,293] (published after the review's search date) were found which addressed the effectiveness of antidepressant therapies versus placebo or active comparator. No controlled trials were found on electroconvulsive therapy or behavioural therapy for the treatment of depression in PD people.

The Cochrane review included three trials: one trial[294] compared a selective serotonin re-uptake inhibitor (SSRI) with placebo; another study[295] compared a tricyclic antidepressant (TCA) with placebo; and the third trial[296] compared the effectiveness of an SSRI versus a TCA.

These trials included small sample sizes (range 22–47). There were several methodological limitations of the included studies: lack of power calculations, lack of baseline characteristics, and no details on methods of randomisation and allocation concealment. The duration of the included trials varied from 16 to 52 weeks (with one study not reporting the trial duration).

One of the independent RCTs[292] compared the effectiveness of an SSRI with placebo. The methodological limitations of this study included unclear methods of randomisation and allocation concealment, small sample size (N=12, six in each arm) and lack of power calculations. The study reported that, because of the low recruitment, the study was terminated after 10 weeks.

The second independent RCT[293] compared repetitive transcranial magnetic stimulation (rTMS) versus an SSRI as an effective antidepressant therapy. The methodological limitations included: short trial duration (8 weeks), small sample size (N=42, 21 in each arm) and lack of power calculation.

▷ Evidence statements

The Cochrane review[291] reported the following non-significant results:

- Nortriptyline (TCA) improved depressive symptoms in the first half of a crossover trial with no deterioration in parkinsonian symptoms.
- Citalopram (SSRI) provided no additional benefit over placebo in the treatment of depressive symptoms in a parallel trial design.
- Fluvoxamine (SSRI) and amitriptyline (TCA) showed similar efficacy in an open-label trial.
- Confusion and visual hallucination were infrequently reported in people taking fluvoxamine and amitriptyline; otherwise, no other major adverse events were reported. (1++)

One of the independent RCTs[293] reported no significant difference between sertraline (SSRI) and placebo in terms of 'response' to treatment (defined as at least 50% reduction of the pre-treatment Montgomery-Asberg Depression Rating Scale), or UPDRS motor scores. (1+)

One of the independent RCTs[292] reported that the following outcomes were improved in both rTMS and fluoxetine-treated groups: the Hamilton Depression Rating Scale and BDI, ADL scores, and the Mini-Mental State Examination (MMSE), with no significant differences between groups. However, adverse events were found more frequently in the fluoxetine-treated group than the rTMS group (p=0.03). (1+)

▷ From evidence to recommendation

There is insufficient evidence from RCTs of the efficacy or safety of any antidepressant therapy in PD. This includes cognitive behavioural therapy, all classes of antidepressant medication and electroconvulsive therapy.

NICE has recently published guidelines[18] for the management of depression which include people with physical disorders. While it is tempting to adopt these guidelines for people with PD, there are a number of factors that suggest that the management of depression in PD may require different strategies:

- There are case reports suggesting that some antidepressants may make PD motor symptoms worse.[297]
- There are established, but rare, interactions between some antidepressants and dopaminergic therapy for PD (eg MAOB inhibitors and antidepressants).[298]
- Cognitive behavioural therapy is not widely available to secondary care teams looking after people with PD.

There is an urgent need for further research to establish effective and safe treatments for depression in PD.

RECOMMENDATIONS

R59   Clinicians should have a low threshold for diagnosing depression in PD.   **D (GPP)**

R60   Clinicians should be aware that there are difficulties in diagnosing mild depression
in people with PD because the clinical features of depression overlap with the motor
features of PD.   **D (GPP)**

R61   The management of depression in people with PD should be tailored to the individual,
in particular, to their co-existing therapy.   **D (GPP)**

9.2.2 Psychotic symptoms

Psychotic symptoms indicate a loss of reality testing; that is, the formation of beliefs and sensations without a basis in reason or external sensory stimulus. Delusions (false unshakeable beliefs that cannot be understood from the individual's sociocultural context) and hallucinations (perceptions in any sensory modality occurring without external sensory stimulus) are the most common symptoms of psychosis.

Psychotic symptoms may occur at any stage in PD. Up to 50% of people with the condition may develop psychotic symptoms[299] and 30% may experience hallucinations within the first 5 years.[300] Although visual hallucination is the most frequent psychotic symptom, a degree of auditory hallucination is found in 40%.[300] Delusions may involve themes of persecution, infidelity and jealousy but these are much less common.

The aetiology of psychotic symptoms in PD is complex. They may arise from the neurotransmitter disturbances of PD but can be caused by any of the drugs used to treat motor symptoms.

The appearance of psychotic symptoms requires careful evaluation. Psychotic symptoms may also occur as part of delirium (caused by other physical illness or drug treatments) or dementia, or may indicate the development of a co-morbid mental illness.

Psychotic symptoms are distressing and may be frightening to people with PD and their carers who may not appreciate that they are symptoms of illness. It is essential to explain the nature of these symptoms to people with PD and their carers.

What is the effectiveness of atypical antipsychotic therapies versus placebo or active comparator in the treatment of psychotic symptoms in PD?

▷ Methodology

Five RCTs[301–305] were found which addressed the effectiveness of atypical antipsychotic therapies versus placebo or active comparator in the treatment of psychosis.

Three trials[306–308] were found that compared two atypical antipsychotic drugs, and these were excluded as within drug class comparisons.

The methodological limitations for some of the included studies involved: lack of randomisation and allocation concealment methods, lack of multi-centre comparative results analysis, lack of power calculations, small sample sizes (N=31[309], 160[303], 30[302] and 60[304]) short trial duration and no intention-to-treat analysis protocols.

▷ Evidence statements

With respect to psychiatric outcomes:

- Trials which looked at the effectiveness of clozapine versus placebo found the following outcomes in favour of active drug treatment:
    - CGI scale (p=0.002)[301], (p=0.001)[304]
    - Brief Psychiatric Rating Scale (BPRS) score (p=0.002)[301]
    - BPRS-Modified score (p=0.003)[301]
    - Scale for the Assessment of Positive Symptoms (p=0.01)[301]
    - Positive and Negative Syndrome Scale positive subscore (p<0.001).[304] (1+)
- Trials which looked at the effectiveness of olanzapine versus placebo found no significant differences between groups on a battery of neuropsychological tests.[302,303] (1+)
- One trial which looked at quetiapine versus placebo found no significant difference between groups on the Baylor PD Hallucination Questionnaire, the BPRDS, and a battery of neuropsychological tests.[305] (1+)

With respect to motor outcomes:

- One trial which looked at clozapine versus placebo reported a beneficial effect of clozapine on UPDRS tremor subscore (p=0.02).[301] (1+)
- Other trials which looked at olanzapine versus placebo reported that the following outcomes worsened with drug treatment:
    - UPDRS total (p=0.007 and p=0.024)[303]
    - UPDRS motor scores (p=0.023 and p=0.039),[303] (p<0.05)[302]
    - subscores gait (p<0.001) and hypokinesia (p<0.05)[302]
    - timed tapping scores (p<0.05)[302]
    - UPDRS ADL scores (p=0.004 and p=0.009).[303] (1+)
- The trial that looked at quetiapine found no differences between placebo and active drug groups on UPDRS ADL or motor scores. There was also no difference found on the Goetz Dyskinesia Rating Scale scores.[305] (1+)

With respect to adverse events:

- The following events were reported as significantly increased in people receiving clozapine treatment:
    - increased mean resting heart rate (p=0.046)[301]
    - increased body weight (p=0.005)[301]
    - increased somnolence (53% vs 18%) and worsening of parkinsonism (21.8% vs 4%) (p values not stated).[304] (1+)
- The following events were reported as significantly increased in people receiving olanzapine treatment:
    - extrapyramidal syndrome (p=0.003)[303]
    - hallucinations (p=0.013)[303]
    - increased salivation (p=0.026)[303]
    - no case of agranulosytosis reported.[304] (1+)
- There were no significant differences in adverse events reported in the study on quetiapine versus placebo. The study did report that no people on the active drug dropped out secondary to related adverse events, which included sedation (N=9, 43%), and subjective worsening in PD (N=4, 19%).[305] (1+)

With respect to withdrawal rates:

- Trials on clozapine efficacy reported that most withdrawals were due to either treatment failure[304] or adverse events.[301] (1+)
- Trials which assessed the effectiveness of olanzapine reported:
  - significantly more people receiving olanzapine discontinued (p=0.029), and mostly due to adverse events (p=0.003), compared with placebo.[303] (1+)
- The trial that assessed quetiapine effectiveness reported no significant differences in withdrawal rates. The study found that 81% of the active drug group completed the study, with four patients withdrawing due to serious unrelated illness or lack of effect and poor compliance. In the placebo group 80% of the participants completed the trial; reasons for withdrawal included unrelated serious illness, resulting in death.[305] (1+)

▷ From evidence to recommendation

Psychosis is a common problem in later PD and can be difficult to manage (Figure 9.1). It may be precipitated by intercurrent illnesses (eg infections), addition of new anti-parkinsonian medication or dementia. Correspondingly, the initial treatment of psychosis should include general medical assessment and treatment of any potential causative factor. Consideration should be given to withdrawal of any recently added medication that may have triggered a psychotic reaction. Drugs that are particularly prone to trigger psychosis, such as anticholinergics, selegiline and amantadine, should be withdrawn first. The patient should be evaluated for a fixed cognitive deficit that might suggest the development of dementia.

For psychosis which does not respond to the above measures, no treatment may be required if psychotic features are not troublesome to the patient or their carers.

In more severe psychosis, antipsychotic medication should be considered. Typical antipsychotics (eg phenothiazines and butyrophenones) are well known to exacerbate PD and should not be used. Various atypical antipsychotics have been evaluated in PD, but only clozapine has a licence for this indication in England and Wales:

Several randomised placebo-controlled trials have shown that clozapine can reduce psychotic symptoms in PD without exacerbating parkinsonian features. However, the use of clozapine requires intensive monitoring to detect the uncommon but potentially life-threatening complication of agranulocytosis. As a result, it is rarely used in PD.

Limited trial evidence suggests that olanzapine is not effective against psychotic features and makes parkinsonian symptoms worse.

There are concerns about the safety of olanzapine and risperidone in elderly people with dementia and risk factors for stroke.[310]

There is no evidence from RCTs of the efficacy and safety of quetiapine as an antipsychotic in PD. However, several trials are ongoing in this area. Quetiapine is thought to be relatively safe and does not require haematological monitoring. As a result, quetiapine has been widely used in PD psychosis.

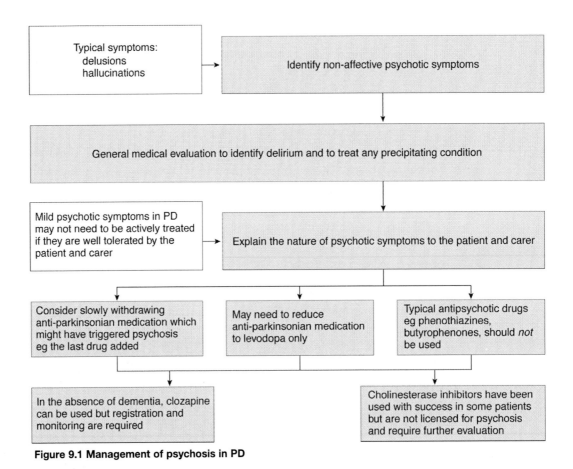

Figure 9.1 Management of psychosis in PD

RECOMMENDATIONS

R62   All people with PD and psychosis should receive a general medical evaluation and treatment for any precipitating condition.   **D (GPP)**

R63   Consideration should be given to withdrawing gradually anti-parkinsonian medication that might have triggered psychosis in people with PD.   **D (GPP)**

R64   Mild psychotic symptoms in people with PD may not need to be actively treated if they are well tolerated by the patient and carer.   **D (GPP)**

R65   Typical antipsychotic drugs (such as phenothiazines and butyrophenones) should not be used in people with PD because they exacerbate the motor features of the condition.   **D (GPP)**

R66   Atypical antipsychotics may be considered for treatment of psychotic symptoms in people with PD, although the evidence base for their efficacy and safety is limited.   **D (GPP)**

R67   Clozapine may be used in the treatment of psychotic symptoms in PD, but registration with a mandatory monitoring scheme is required. It is recognised that few specialists caring for people with PD have experience with clozapine.   **B**

9.2.3 Dementia

PD is associated with impairment of cognitive function. Compared with people without PD, deficits in visuospatial abilities, category learning, verbal fluency, set switching and executive functions are typically reported.

Particular attention has focused on deficits of executive function that may mediate many of the other impairments. Executive functions include working memory, mental flexibility, and the ability to initiate and suppress responses.

Dementia (the progressive loss of global cognitive function) is also common in PD; 48%[305] to 80%[311] of people may develop dementia at some point in the course of the condition.

In addition to cognitive decline, dementia leads to impairment in activities of daily living and disturbance of behaviour and other psychological functions. Dementia in PD is accompanied by reduced quality of life for people with PD and their carers.[290,312]

Other pathologies commonly causing dementia include Alzheimer's disease, vascular brain disease and dementia with Lewy bodies.

Traditionally, dementia developing more than 1 year after the onset of the motor features of PD is referred to as PD with dementia (PDD). Dementia developing within 1 year of the onset of motor features is classified as dementia with Lewy bodies. The relationship between PDD and dementia with Lewy bodies is unclear, but many consider them to be a continuum rather than discrete entities.

Since people with dementia with Lewy bodies may not develop parkinsonism, we have not considered the treatment of this type of dementia in this guideline. The GDG acknowledges that this decision may need to be revisited in the future if new evidence proves that a continuum exists between PDD and dementia with Lewy bodies.

Rarely, dementia may arise due to a treatable illness. All people with dementia require careful evaluation of their medical condition, treatment and investigations to clarify the diagnosis with attention to potentially treatable conditions. In this context, cognitive decline due to depression, often referred to as depressive 'pseudodementia', should be considered.

The assessment and management of dementia will require a range of clinical expertise that can be provided only by a multidisciplinary team.

Are cholinesterase inhibitors effective cognitive enhancement therapies in PD?

▷ Methodology

Seven papers[313–319] were found which addressed the effectiveness of cholinesterase inhibitors as cognitive enhancement therapies in PD. All levels of evidence (RCTs and case series) were selected in order to provide a comprehensive body of evidence upon which to analyse the cost-effectiveness of these treatments in people with PDD. In addition, the literature search cut-off date, for this particular section of the guideline, was August 2005 instead of February 2005.

In addition to the seven papers selected, a Cochrane review[320] which included only one RCT[321] on rivastigmine versus placebo was excluded. This paper was excluded as the patient population was defined as people suffering from dementia with Lewy bodies and not PDD.

▷ Evidence statements

Table 9.1 Effectiveness of cholinesterase inhibitors for people with PDD (1++)				
	Rivastigmine		**Donepezil**	**Galantamine**
Study design	RCT	CS	RCT	CS
Level of evidence	1++	3	1+	3
Number of trials	1	1	3	1
Sample size (N=)	541[313]	28[318]	22[316], 14[317], 15[314]	16[319]
Trial duration (weeks)	24[313]	34[318]	10[316,317], 16[314]	8[319]
Key cognitive outcomes				
ADAS-cog	C[313]	C[318]	NS[316], NR[317], NR[314],	NR[319]
MMSE	C[313]	NS[318]	C[316], C[317], NS[314]	NS[319]
Motor outcomes				
UPDRS total	NR[313]	NS[318]	NS[316], NS[317], NR[314]	NR[319]
UPDRS motor	NS[313]	NS[318]	NS[316], NS[317], NR[314]	NR[319]

CS = case series; RCT = randomised controlled trial; NR = not reported; NS = not statistically significant (p>0.05); C = statistically significantly (p<0.05) in favour of treatment with cholinesterase inhibition; P = statistically significantly (p<0.05) in favour of placebo treatment.

Other cognitive outcomes reported to be in favour (p<0.05) of cholinesterase inhibitor treatment:

- Neuropsychiatric Inventory 10[313]
- Alzheimer's disease assessment scale (ADAS-cog)[313]
- Alzheimer's Disease Cooperative Study (ADCS)-CGIC[313]
- ADCS ADL[313]
- Cognitive Drug Research power of attention tests[313]
- Delis-Kaplan Executive Function System[*][313]
- Ten-point clock-drawing test[313]
- Dementia Rating Scale memory subscore[314]
- CGI[316] (1++)
- Clinical impression of change at weeks 12 and 26[318]
- UPDRS subscore part I (mental)[318]
- Clock-drawing test.[319] (3)

Other cognitive outcomes reported to be improved in people treated with galantamine:[319]

- Hallucinations improved in 78% of people who experienced hallucinations at baseline.
- Cognition improved in 62% of people and declined in 31%.[319] (3)

---

*Because executive function tests were not performed at all sites, these tests included only people who actually took these tests (74% and 18% of patient population respectively).

A third case series study[315] reported the following outcomes specific to the trial's PDD population:

- In people diagnosed with PDD there was an association with increased probability of an MMSE response (p=0.02).
- PDD patients improved by a mean of 2.3 MMSE points. (3)

With respect to adverse events:

- In the rivastigmine-treatment group:
  - More adverse events were experienced (p<0.001).[313]
  - Parkinsonian symptoms were more frequent (p=0.002).[313]
  - The most common events included: tremor (p=0.01), nausea and vomiting (p<0.001). (1++)
  - 40% of people had to decrease the daily dose.[318] (3)
- In the donepezil-treatment group:
  - There was a non-significant difference in incidence.[314]
  - Events leading to withdrawal included: constipation, nausea and vomiting, hypersalivation, worsening of motor symptoms (gait impairment, increased number of falls, increased tremor).[314,317] (1+)
- In the galantamine-treatment group:[319]
  - Three people withdrew prematurely due to vomiting, worsening tremor, anorexia and nausea. (3)

With respect to withdrawals:

- There was no significant difference in rivastigmine trials.[313,320] (1+)
- The donepezil-treatment group remained in the trial 4.2 weeks longer on average (p<0.05).[314]
- 57% of donepezil group versus 11% of placebo group withdrew due to adverse events.[314] (1+)

▷ From evidence to recommendation

There is evidence from randomised placebo-controlled trials of the effectiveness and safety of cholinesterase inhibitors in the treatment of PDD. They are effective in treating both cognitive decline and psychosis in this context. However, not all patients respond, so regular review of the need for these agents is required.

At the time of writing, only one of the cholinesterase inhibitors has a product licence in the UK. The GDG considers that these are useful agents that are commonly used in clinical practice and that they should be available.

NICE has commissioned the guideline: 'Dementia: management of dementia, including use of antipsychotic medication in older people'. NICE is developing this guideline in collaboration with the Social Care Institute for Excellence. This guideline will cover all major forms of dementia, including Alzheimer's disease, vascular dementia, Lewy body dementia, subcortical dementia, frontotemporal dementias, and mixed cortical and subcortical dementia. Dementia encountered in the course of PD will be addressed. The guidelines will, where appropriate, address the differences in treatment and care for people with mild, moderate and severe dementia.

RECOMMENDATION

R68   Although cholinesterase inhibitors have been used successfully in individual people
with PD dementia, further research is recommended to identify those patients who will
benefit from this treatment.   **D (GPP)**

9.3   Sleep disturbance

*'He has lots and lots of nightmares when he goes to sleep, and he
comes to and doesn't know where he is...'*   (carer)[2]

Sleep problems are common in PD and comprise:

- daytime hypersomnolence
- nocturnal akinesia
- restless leg syndrome (RLS) (Ekbom's syndrome)
- periodic leg movements of sleep
- REM sleep behaviour disorder (RBD)
- sudden onset of sleep
- vivid dreams and/or hallucinations
- nocturia (passing of urine frequently – three times or more – at night)
- sleep fragmentation.

They are particularly taxing to people with PD and their bed-partners because of their
mixed nature comprising motor, sensory and sleep issues. In addition, if inadequate rest is
gained by night, there is a high prevalence of excessive daytime somnolence that may have
serious consequences on social functioning and safety.[322]

Assessment should include a thorough sleep history including:

- enquiry about the three phases of sleep: initiation, maintenance and awakening
- enquiry about leg movements – periodic leg movements in sleep, RLS
- hallucinations and vivid dreams
- questioning whether dreams are acted out, sometimes violently, indicative of RBD, which
  occurs in up to 15% of people with PD and may precede the diagnosis of PD.

Drug-induced hallucinations and/or vivid dreams may occur, and should be distinguished from
RBD. Many centrally acting drugs may disturb sleep patterns, mainly by inducing sedation, but
some may cause nocturnal alertness (eg selegiline).

One of the most common sleep disorders seen in PD is RLS. The International RLS Study
Group[323] criteria for the diagnosis of RLS are:

- desire to move the extremities, usually associated with discomfort or disagreeable
  sensations in the extremities
- motor restlessness – people move to relieve the discomfort (eg walking, or providing a
  counter-stimulus to relieve the discomfort such as rubbing the legs)
- symptoms are worse at rest with at least temporary relief by activity
- symptoms are worse later in the day or at night.

Vivid dreams and nightmares may be provoked by many of the commonly used drugs in PD. A review of medication and reduction/avoidance of suspected causes is usually effective. However, RBD may also occur in which dreams are so vivid that they are acted out. When pharmacotherapy is required, a response may be seen to low doses of clonazepam.[322]

'Sudden onset of sleep' without warning has recently been described in PD people, with the potential to cause road traffic accidents.[324] While certain dopamine agonists were initially incriminated, current opinion is that all PD medications can cause daytime hypersomnolence and that all people with PD are liable to hypersomnolence and should be warned of the possibility of falling asleep at the wheel. This may be more likely in people with later PD on multiple medications and also during upwards dose titration, particularly with dopaminergic agonists. Any people so affected should not drive.

RECOMMENDATIONS

R69   A full sleep history should be taken from people with PD who report sleep
        disturbance.   D (GPP)

R70   Good sleep hygiene should be advised in people with PD with any sleep disturbance and
        includes:
        - avoidance of stimulants (for example coffee, tea, caffeine) in the evening
        - establishment of a regular pattern of sleep
        - comfortable bedding and temperature
        - provision of assistive devices, such as a bed lever or rails to aid with moving and turning,
          allowing the person to get more comfortable
        - restriction of daytime siestas
        - advice about taking regular and appropriate exercise to induce better sleep
        - a review of all medication and avoidance of any drugs that may affect sleep or
          alertness, or may interact with other medication (for example, selegiline,
          antihistamines, H_2 antagonists, antipsychotics and sedatives).   D (GPP)

R71   Care should be taken to identify and manage restless leg syndrome (RLS) and rapid
        eye movement (REM) sleep behaviour disorder in people with PD and sleep
        disturbance.   D (GPP)

R72   People with PD who have sudden onset of sleep should be advised not to drive and
        to consider any occupational hazards. Attempts should be made to adjust their
        medication to reduce its occurrence.   D (GPP)

9.3.1 Daytime hypersomnolence

It has been recognised in recent years that daytime hypersomnolence is a major issue for people with PD. This may even lead to the sudden onset of sleep, which can be dangerous.

How effective is modafinil in treating daytime hypersomnolence in PD?

▷ Methodology

Three placebo-controlled, double-blind RCTs[325,326,327] were found which investigated the effectiveness of modafinil treatment for sleep disorders in people with PD. Two of the studies used a 200 mg/d dose[325,326] while the third increased the dose to 400 mg/d after 1 week.[327]

All studies were small (N=15, 21 and 40)[325,326,327] and of short duration (between 4 and 8 weeks). The mean age of the people included in these studies was 65 years, with mean disease duration of 7 years.

No RCTs were found on the specific treatment of RBD and RLS in PD.

▷ Evidence statements

With respect to the Epworth Sleepiness Scale (ESS):
- One study[325] demonstrated the change in ESS was statistically significant in favour of modafinil treatment (95% CI −8.6 to −0.2, p=0.039). (1+)
- Another study[327] found no significant change in ESS between modafinil and placebo groups. (1++)

With respect to patient-rated scales:
- The patient-rated CGI scale improved significantly on modafinil (p=0.07).[325] (1+)
- There was no difference between modafinil and placebo groups in terms of change in sleepiness 'much or very much improved'.[327] (1++)

With respect to other outcome measures:
- There were *no* significant differences between modafinil and placebo in the largest study[327] for the following:
    - UPDRS ADL and motor scores
    - Multiple sleep latency test
    - SF-36
    - Fatigue Severity Scale
    - Hamilton depression scale
    - adverse events
    - withdrawal rates. (1++)
- There were *no* significant differences between modafinil and placebo for the following in the two smaller studies:[325,326]
    - Maintenance of Wakefulness Test[326]
    - mean changes in sleep latency[326]
    - sleep logs (similar amounts of sleep)[326]
    - Beck depression scores[326]
    - physician-rated CGIC[325]
    - worsening/improvement of PD signs[325]
    - UPDRS scores, Hoehn and Yahr scores, timed tapping tests or patient diaries[325]
    - percentage on time[325]
    - adverse events[325,326]
    - withdrawal rates.[325,326] (1+)

▷ From evidence to recommendation

While there is little evidence from RCTs of the efficacy and safety of modafinil in the treatment of daytime hypersomnolence in PD, it has a product licence for use in hypersomnolence in chronic diseases. Members of the GDG have little experience in its use but acknowledged that modafinil can be useful in this clinical context.

RECOMMENDATION

R73 Modafinil may be considered for daytime hypersomnolence in people with PD. **D (GPP)**

9.3.2 Nocturnal akinesia

Turning over in bed (nocturnal akinesia) may become difficult in PD due to truncal rigidity. This can have a major impact on people with PD and can interfere with sleep and thus lead to daytime hypersomnolence.

Treatment has traditionally been with either small doses of immediate-release levodopa or controlled-release levodopa last thing at night. There is insufficient experience with dopamine agonists and COMT inhibitors in this area.

Are controlled-release levodopa preparations effective in the management of nocturnal akinesia in PD?

▷ Methodology

A double-blind RCT[328] was found which compared controlled-release levodopa and immediate-release levodopa in the treatment of nocturnal and early-morning disability.

The RCT was a multi-centre trial including 103 people from 11 centres in the UK. The mean age of people included in the study was 68 years, with average disease duration of 8 years. Controlled-release co-beneldopa or immediate-release co-beneldopa was given at a dose of 125 mg/day immediately before going to bed.

Methodological limitations included: lack of randomisation and allocation concealment methods, no washout period or first-arm results, and intention-to-treat analysis was not stated. However, carry-over effects and differences between centres were statistically analysed and produced no significant differences.

▷ Evidence statements

With respect to controlled-release levodopa versus immediate-release levodopa, one study[328] reported the following outcomes:
- There were no significant differences in nocturnal and early morning disability. (1+)

▷ From evidence to recommendation

There is insufficient evidence from RCTs to support the use of controlled-release levodopa preparations in the treatment of nocturnal akinesia in PD. However, the GDG had considerable experience of their use in this context and were able to support their value.

There is also some experience in using long-acting dopamine agonists, especially cabergoline, for nocturnal akinesia, although such ergot-derived agonists are used less frequently in view of the risk of serosal reactions.

RECOMMENDATION

R74   Modified-release levodopa preparations may be used for nocturnal akinesia in
people with PD.   D (GPP)

9.4   Falls

Falls are common in PD; two-thirds of people with PD fall each year, with most eventually becoming fallers.[12,329,330]

Early onset of falls may indicate an alternative diagnosis to idiopathic PD such as PSP.[331]

Predictors of falls specific to PD include:[12,329,330,332]

- longer disease duration
- more advanced disease
- dyskinesia
- motor fluctuations
- atypical parkinsonism
- postural instability
- small steps
- freezing
- stride-to-stride variability
- altered step and stance width
- loss of arm swing.

Predictors of falls in PD similar to those in the general population include:[12,333]

- old age
- previous falls
- use of sedative drugs
- depression
- dementia.

The clinical impact of falls is considerable, often leading to injury requiring healthcare services, an incapacitating fear of renewed falls, anxiety and depression.[334] The associated costs for society are substantial in terms of finances as well as stress on the patient and their support network.

9.4.1   Assessment and prevention of falls

People with PD require a multidisciplinary assessment of the specific and non-specific predictors of falls together with the intrinsic and extrinsic factors that contribute to falls. In common with other people with repeated falls the assessment and prevention of falls in PD requires multifactorial assessment and intervention by a professional with understanding of PD. The NICE clinical guideline no. 21 'Falls: assessment and prevention of falls in older people'[16] provides a framework for this process. The 'Quick Reference Guide'[335] (Appendix D) of this guideline is applicable to all people with PD.

RECOMMENDATION

R75   For all people with PD at risk of falling, please refer to *Falls: assessment and prevention of falls in older people*. NICE clinical guideline no. 21. (Available from **www.nice.org.uk/CG021**) (**NICE 2004**)

9.5   Autonomic disturbance

Autonomic dysfunction is common in PD due to the underlying pathophysiology of the condition affecting the catecholaminergic neurones of the autonomic nervous system.

While symptoms due to autonomic disturbance are common, and while this area has not undergone a systematic search for treatment trials, several crucial issues specific to PD were identified by the GDG as Good Practice Points.

9.5.1   Gastrointestinal dysfunction

▷   Weight loss

Unintended weight loss is common in PD, occurring in over 50% of individuals, with 20% losing over 12 kg in one study.[336] A larger proportion of women than men with PD may experience weight loss. Moderate or severe dyskinesia is the strongest correlate of under-nutrition in PD, although the reasons for weight loss are likely to be more complex than simply 'burning off' more calories.[337] Similarly, the weight gain commonly observed after bilateral DBS has not yet been adequately explained.

When significant weight loss occurs, the following general points should be considered:
- other medical causes for weight loss (eg malignancy, endocrine causes)
- investigation of swallow[338]
- review of anti-parkinsonian medications if dyskinesias are problematic
- dietary supplements
- referral to a dietitian.

▷   Dysphagia

Dysphagia is an impairment of swallowing. It is a complex process with risks of asphyxiation, aspiration pneumonia, malnutrition and dehydration. Swallowing difficulties in PD usually relate to disease severity and may affect all phases of the swallow process (oral, pharyngeal and oesophageal). Abnormalities are often detected on video fluoroscopy (modified barium swallow).

One group[339] studied 75 people at different stages of PD and showed that up to 94% had problems with swallowing. In Hoehn and Yahr stages I–III the problems were often not noticed by the person with PD. However, abnormalities are often detected on modified barium swallow testing. In advanced PD, swallowing difficulties can be severe and are usually obvious to patients and their carers. There is a high incidence of silent aspiration in PD,[340] putting the person at risk of developing recurrent chest infections if not properly investigated. Infected oral secretions are a prime cause of pneumonia and this may be caused by poor oral hygiene due to reduced motor movement in the mouth. Pneumonia is a leading cause of death in later stages of PD.[341]

Dysphagia in PD results from catecholaminergic degeneration and Lewy body formation in the brainstem and within the pharyngeal muscles. It does not respond fully to optimisation of dopaminergic medication.[342]

Dysphagia poses a major problem to the taking of medications which are critical in the successful management of PD. Reduced tongue control leads to difficulty manipulating and clearing tablets from the mouth. Pharyngeal pooling and dysmotility may lead to retention of pills in the valleculae and pyriform fossae; consequently, delivery of medications may be erratic.

The management of dysphagia in PD may involve the following generic issues:
- There should be early referral to a speech and language therapist for assessment, swallowing advice and, where indicated, further instrumental investigation (eg videofluoroscopy or fibreoptic endoscopic examination of swallow safety (FEES)).
- Videofluoroscopy/FEES should be considered to exclude silent aspiration.
- The problems associated with eating and swallowing should be managed on a case-by-case basis. Problems should be anticipated and supportive measures employed to prevent complications where possible.
- Enteral feeding options may need to be considered. This may involve short-term nasogastric tube feeding to re-establish a suitable drug regimen, or placement of a longer-term feeding system such as a percutaneous endoscopic gastrostomy.
- Cricopharyngeal (CP) myotomy has been reported to be successful in some cases with specific CP deficits. However, treatment must be based on physiology, which is best revealed with videofluoroscopy. CP myotomy may put people with PD at high risk of laryngeal penetration and pulmonary aspiration if oral and pharyngeal dysphagia is present.[343,344] CP myotomy also puts people at high risk of aspiration of reflux from the stomach.

▷ Constipation

Colonic dysmotility and anorectal dysfunction are common in PD, occurring in up to 30% and 60% of cases, respectively.[345] Lewy body degeneration occurs within the myenteric plexus of the colon in PD, leading to slow transit times and, occasionally, megacolon, intestinal pseudo-obstruction and volvulus. A combination of disordered contraction and relaxation of the muscles of defecation, which may in part be dystonic, leads to excessive straining, pain, and a sense of incomplete evacuation. Faecal incontinence, when it occurs in PD, is usually due to overflow around faecal impaction.

The management of constipation due to colonic dysmotility in PD should follow a staged, or stepladder, approach:[345]
- increasing dietary fibre and fluid intake (at least eight glasses of water per day) and avoiding bananas

- increasing exercise
- fibre supplements such as psyllium[346] or methylcellulose
- stool softener (eg docusate)
- osmotic laxative (eg lactulose)
- polyethylene glycol electrolyte-balanced solutions[347]
- occasional enemas when required.

For further details on nutrition support in adults, please refer to the NICE guideline on 'Nutrition support in adults' available from **www.nice.org.uk/page.aspx?o=292900**

▷ Genitourinary dysfunction

Urinary dysfunction

Up to 75% of people with PD develop bladder problems. Nocturia is the earliest and most common urinary problem, although daytime urgency and frequency may also be troublesome. Urinary incontinence is common in PD. Detrusor overactivity of neurogenic origin appears to result from disinhibition of the ponto-mesencephalic micturition centre.[348]

Where there are refractory or persistent bladder problems, referral to a person with urological expertise should be considered.

Other management approaches include:
- excluding urinary tract infection where there is an abrupt change in voiding pattern
- excluding diabetes mellitus where frequency and polyuria are prominent
- use of anticholinergic agents (tolterodine, oxybutynin, propiverine, solifenacin), although, since these drugs cross the blood-brain barrier, they must be used with caution as they may induce a toxic confusional state. Other drugs may be available which do not cross the blood-brain barrier (eg trospium chloride).

▷ Sexual dysfunction

Erectile dysfunction is more common in PD (60–70%) than in age-matched controls (38%).[349,350] Men with PD may also experience sexual dissatisfaction and premature ejaculation. In women, difficulties with arousal, low sexual desire and anorgasmia are common.[349]

Dopaminergic therapy may also induce hypersexuality, even when there is erectile dysfunction.

In the management of erectile dysfunction the following should be considered:
- co-morbid endocrine abnormalities (eg hypothyroidism, hyperprolactinaemia)
- 'latent' depression
- discontinuation of drugs associated with erectile dysfunction (eg alpha-blockers) or anorgasmia (eg SSRIs)
- type V cGMP-specific phosphodiesterase inhibitors (eg sildenafil)
- intracavernous injections or transurethral suppositories of alprostadil (a synthetic prostaglandin E_1).

9.5.2 Orthostatic hypotension

Orthostatic hypotension (OH) occurs in 48% of people with PD in the community[351] but is asymptomatic in up to 60%.[352] It may be defined as a drop in systolic blood pressure after standing greater than or equal to 20 mmHg or to less than 90 mmHg.[353] The aetiology of OH in PD is multifactorial and includes Lewy body degeneration in the hypothalamus, brainstem and peripheral nervous system. Symptoms of OH include fatigue, pre-syncope and syncope, while OH may also contribute to falling. Persisting or troublesome OH may warrant referral to a unit with expertise in falls and syncope.

The management of OH in PD should follow a stepladder approach:

- eliminate or reduce antihypertensive medications; reduce or change anti-parkinsonian drugs
- increase dietary salt and fluid intake, avoid caffeine at night; eat frequent, small meals and avoid alcohol
- elevate head of bed by 30–40°
- salt-retaining steroid (eg fludrocortisone)
- direct-acting sympathomimetic (eg midodrine, only available on named-patient basis).

9.5.3 Excessive sweating

Severe sweating may occur as an end-of-dose off phenomenon or while in the on motor state, usually associated with dyskinesias.

The management approach to excessive sweating should exclude a comorbid medical problem (eg chronic infection, thyrotoxicosis), or the post-menopausal state.

9.5.4 Sialorrhoea

Excessive saliva or drooling occurs in 70–80% of people with PD and may be more common in men.[354,355] It may result from oropharyngeal dysfunction, including reduced swallow frequency. Apart from social embarrassment and soiling of clothing, sialorrhoea may also be associated with perioral infection.

General management measures may include:

- referral to a speech and language therapist for full assessment of swallowing ability
- advice and trial of behavioural management techniques to encourage regular saliva swallows
- use of a portable metronomic brooch as a reminder for saliva swallows[356]
- lip seal and swallow exercises
- sublingual 1% atropine ophthalmic solution twice daily[357]
- injection of salivary glands with botulinum toxin A.[358]

RECOMMENDATION

R76   People with PD should be treated appropriately for the following autonomic
         disturbances: D (GPP)

* urinary dysfunction
* weight loss
* dysphagia
* constipation
* erectile dysfunction
* orthostatic hypotension
* excessive sweating
* sialorrhoea.

9.6   Pain

Pain is defined as an unpleasant or distressing sensory experience.[359] Pain occurs in around
40% of people with PD but is rarely a major feature of the disorder.

Pain in PD has been classified[359] as:

* musculoskeletal – often secondary to parkinsonian rigidity and hypokinesia (eg frozen
  shoulder)
* dystonic – associated with dystonic movements and postures which often occur in the off
  period in the feet
* primary or central – burning or paraesthetic pain outwith a dermatome or root territory
  which is not explained by a musculoskeletal or dystonic cause
* neuropathic – pain in the distribution of a root or nerve with associated signs
* akathisia-related – inner feeling of restlessness leading to inability to keep still.

Little research has been done in this area and the management of many of these types of pain is
generic rather than being specific to PD. Therefore, the GDG elected not to undertake a
literature search in this area. The GDG did recognise the importance of dystonic pain which is
often responsive to dopaminergic medications (see Chapter 7).

10 | Other key interventions

'Never has anybody said to us, "Do you think you need a physiotherapist, a speech therapist, or an occupational therapist – do you need these services?" That's something we have gone out to find ourselves and I think too late.' (carer)[2]

10.1 Introduction

In previous chapters, consideration has been given to the evidence for pharmacological treatments and surgical interventions. People with PD may also benefit from interventions provided by a range of health disciplines. This chapter addresses the effectiveness of specific interventions that are part of:

- PD specialist nursing
- physiotherapy
- occupational therapy
- speech and language therapy.

Because service issues lie outside the scope of this guideline, evidence has been sought for the effectiveness of the interventions that are part of a discipline and recommendations made accordingly. It should be noted that some interventions, particularly those related to maintaining independence, may, in practice, be carried out by professionals from a number of disciplines.

10.1.1 Methodological limitations

When reviewing the evidence of the interventions delivered by health professionals the following methodological limitations should be considered:

- variations in location of therapy (home, outpatient clinic, in hospital)
- lack of reporting the intensity of therapy given
- variations in therapy regimen between trials
- unclear qualifications and experience of person delivering the intervention
- short trial duration and lack of long-term follow-up
- small sample sizes without power calculations provided
- lack of reporting methods of randomisation or allocation concealment
- lack of reporting drop-outs from trials
- lack of intention-to-treat analysis.

10.2 Parkinson's disease nurse specialist interventions

PDNS care has been pioneered in the UK over the last 10 years supported by the UK PDS. A PDNS's role is defined[360] as a specialist practitioner with essential skills in:

- communication (see Appendix C)
- patient and carer assessment

- symptom management
- medicines management
- providing ongoing support and advice
- referral to other therapists
- education.

A recent report from the UK PDS (2004)[361] identified the key roles and responsibilities of the PDNS in the UK as:

- making and receiving referrals directly to create an integrated and responsive service for people with PD
- admitting and discharging people for specified conditions and within agreed protocols
- managing caseloads
- providing information, education and support to people in their homes, in clinics and in hospitals
- prescribing medicines and treatment and monitoring the effectiveness of changes in medication and treatment
- using the latest information technology (IT) to triage people with PD to the most appropriate health professional
- using IT to identify people at risk and speed up responses to crises.

What is the effectiveness of PDNS care versus standard medical care in the management of people with PD?

10.2.1 Methodology

Three RCTs[362,363,364] were found which addressed the effectiveness of PDNS or other non-consultant care. The specific intervention of 'nursing care', the comparator and the sample size varied between the studies limiting the ability to draw general conclusions. The three studies and their variables are listed below:

- the effects of community-based PDNS care versus GP care in 1869 people with PD[362]
- the effects of nurse practitioner care versus 'standard care' in a population of 40 people with PD recruited from a specialist neurology unit[363]
- the effects of substituted consultant care versus PDNS care in a population of 185 people with PD attending hospital clinics.[364]

Only one study provided data on statistical power.[362] Another study[364] involved only 58% of the 185 enrolled participants who completed the trial, and in a third study[363] the sample size was small (N=40).

The study environment varied considerably between trials. In one study,[362] 438 GP practices were involved from nine randomly selected English health authorities. The practices recruited people who represented the PD population of England and Wales. In another study,[364] clinics in London and Hull with established PDNS services were selected to participate. This study had large numbers of crossovers (ie people receiving care from both consultants and PDNSs), which makes interpretation difficult. Finally, a third study[363] considered only people recruited from the National Hospital for Neurology and Neurosurgery in London. The lack of random patient and centre selection methods in the latter studies limits their generalisability to care provided elsewhere in the UK.

10.2.2 Health economic methodology

Three economic studies of PDNS care were critically appraised[362,364,365] and one met quality criteria.[362] One study[364] did not meet quality criteria in the health economic analysis, but was included in the clinical efficacy analysis. The reason for the exclusion here is due to a 42% loss of people during follow-up, which may have led to bias in the economic results. The third study[365] was also excluded as the trial did not consider all costs relevant to the provision of PDNS care to reflect true cost-saving estimates.

The one study[362] that met quality criteria evaluated community-based PDNS care with GP care versus standard GP care in an RCT in the UK.

As part of the guideline development process, we have evaluated the cost-effectiveness of PDNS care in comparison to standard care over a 1-year period from the NHS perspective. Full details of this analysis are shown in Appendix G.

10.2.3 Evidence statements

The PDNS versus GP care study[362] evaluated the results of the Global Health Questionnaire at the end of a 2-year period and found only one significant outcome measure (out of approximately 20 measures) which favoured PDNS care (treatment difference –0.23, 95% CI –0.4 to –0.06, p=0.008). (1+)

This study also reported non-significant results for the following outcome measures: 2-year and 4-year mortality, stand-up tests, bone fracture, mean best hand score, EuroQol tariff, dot-in-square score, PDQ-39 measures, physical functioning (SF-36) and general health (SF-36). (1+)

The trial also found that PDNS care enabled more rapid implementation of what was then thought to be good prescribing practice:

- The proportion of people with PD taking controlled-release levodopa increased significantly more in the nurse group (p=0.016).
- People in the nurse group had a greater tendency after 2 years to discontinue their use of selegiline (p<0.001).[362] (1+)
- After 1 year, another trial[364] found that substituted consultant care produced the following outcomes (out of 22 measures):
  - one significant outcome in favour of PDNS care: the communication score on the PDQ-39 questionnaire (p=0.05)
  - two significant outcomes favouring the consultant care group: physical functioning on SF-36 (p=0.02) and general health on SF-36 (p=0.02). (1+)
- The nurse practitioner versus standard care RCT[363] assessed people with PD and dystonia over 6 months. For the psychosocial outcome measures, no significant differences were found between the intervention and control groups. (1+)

In addition, the results from an independent assessment[363] of patient satisfaction, in just the intervention group arm, showed that:

- The most common information provided by the nursing intervention concerned practical issues such as income support and mobility allowance.
- The mean rating for the nursing intervention was 8.5 on a scale of 1–10 (one-half rated the contact as 10, ie 'very useful').

- The aspect of the intervention most highly ranked in terms of usefulness was 'the opportunity to talk to someone about the illness and the problems caused by it'.
- 89% considered the home visits the most useful aspect of the intervention.
- 81% thought that the duration of contact with the PDNS needed to be prolonged.
- 58% thought that the PDNS intervention would be useful to other people with PD (mean 9.0 on scale of 1–10). (3)

10.2.4 Health economic evidence statements

The RCT[362] found no significant difference in mean increase in annual costs between groups (p=0.47) from the year before the study to the second year of the study. This mean annual cost estimated the provision of nurse specialist care to cost £200 per person per year and excluded the cost of apomorphine. The mean annual cost in the specialist nurse group increased from £4,050 to £5,860 (£ 1996) and from £3,480 to £5,630 in the control group based on 1,859 people from 438 general practices in nine randomly selected health authority areas of England.

It is not always clear whether PDNS care is substituting some or all of the consultant care or is serving as additional care.[364] By varying the cost-savings of other health professional costs by PDNS care, costs for 1 year of PDNS care range from an additional cost of £3,289 to cost-savings of £4,564. Full details of these analyses are shown in Appendix G.

10.2.5 From evidence to recommendation

Most of the benefits derived from PDNS interventions have been shown to relate to the overall patient care experience and the delivery of services such as the monitoring of medication and provision of information. The communication issues for people with PD and their carers are further addressed in Chapter 4.

There has only been limited evidence showing improvements in direct measures of outcome.

The evidence indicates the cost-effectiveness of PDNS care is inconclusive.

RECOMMENDATION

R77   People with PD should have regular access to the following: C
- clinical monitoring and medication adjustment
- a continuing point of contact for support, including home visits when appropriate
- a reliable source of information about clinical and social matters of concern to people with PD and their carers,

which may be provided by a Parkinson's disease nurse specialist.

10.3 Physiotherapy

Physiotherapy or physical therapy can be defined as: 'A health care profession which emphasises the use of physical approaches in the promotion, maintenance and restoration of an individual's physical, psychological and social well-being, encompassing variations in health status'.[366]

Physiotherapy primarily addresses the physical components of rehabilitation, essentially to maximise the functional capacity of a person and their role within society.

Where people receiving physiotherapy have a longer-term condition, such as PD, physiotherapy is generally regarded as an active, ongoing process and one that should be client-focused in its approach and regularly reviewed.

Physiotherapy might incorporate only education and advice ensuring maintenance of a current level of fitness and ability, or involve exercises specific to the needs of the person with PD to regain movement, prevent falls, maximise respiratory function or reduce pain. It also has a role alongside medical and surgical intervention to enhance the person's potential with these interventions.

In addition to physiotherapy, other physical adjuncts to therapy may include approaches such as the Alexander Technique, yoga, Conductive Education or Pilates – techniques which not only promote movement, but also are linked with social well-being.

The principles of physiotherapy are:[367]

- early implementation of exercise programme to prevent de-conditioning and other preventable complications
- utilisation of a meaningful and practical assessment procedure to allow monitoring and identification of rehabilitation priorities
- the identification of deterioration and timely, appropriate intervention
- the opportunity for targeted therapy for restoration or compensation of function
- the involvement of patients and carers in decision-making and management strategies.

What is the effectiveness of physiotherapy interventions versus standard therapy in the care of people with PD?

10.3.1 Methodology

A Cochrane systematic review[368] and an RCT[369] were found which addressed the effectiveness of physiotherapy versus standard therapy or placebo in the treatment of PD. Another study[370] was found which addressed the effectiveness of the Alexander Technique versus no therapy or massage therapy.

The physiotherapy RCT[369] (N=8) investigated the effect of a 16-week aerobic exercise programme on aerobic capacity and movement initiation time for PD.

The Alexander Technique RCT[370] (N=88) randomised participants to three groups: controls (N=30) or Alexander Technique (N=29) or massage group (N=29). The massage group received two massage sessions per week for 12 weeks (the massage group was used as control for touch and attention). The Alexander Technique consisted of two 40-minute lessons per week for 12 weeks, then 5 weeks after completion the participants received a short audio tape that led them through a 20-minute lying down exercise.

The Cochrane review[368] included 11 randomised trials; four of these trials[371–374] reported significant outcomes in relation to physiotherapy treatment for people with PD, with a total of 280 people. The participants in these trials received physiotherapy directed to trunk and limb functions and were treated for 8–30 hours over 3–52 weeks. The method of physiotherapy was usually described in a very broad manner; even the time spent by the therapist with the patient was not specified in half of these trials.

10.3.2 Evidence statements

For a summary of the effectiveness of physiotherapy techniques see Table 10.1 below.

Table 10.1 Effectiveness of physiotherapy techniques (1+)			
Outcomes	**(N)**	**Follow-up**	**p value**
Conventional physiotherapy techniques			
Activities of daily living[374]			
Barthel Index	20	Post-intervention	0.05
		5 months	0.045
NUDS		Post-intervention	NS
		5 months	0.018
Functional Index Measure		Post-intervention	0.048
		5 months	0.016
Clinical rating scales			
Total UPDRS[374]	20	Post-intervention	<0.001
		5 months	<0.001
Webster rating scale[374]		Post-intervention	NS
		5 months	0.011
Parkinson's Home Visiting Assessment Tool (5/53 items)[373]	30	8 months	<0.05
Motor impairments			
Walking velocity[372,374]	44	Post-intervention	≤0.002
		5 months	0.006
Stride length[372,374]		Post-intervention	≤0.016
		5 months	0.044
Spinal rotation[371]	51	Post-intervention	0.019
Exercise outcomes[369]			
Aerobic capacity	8	Post-intervention vs controls	0.013
Power output		Post-intervention vs controls	0.037
Movement initiation		Post-intervention vs controls	0.003

continued

Outcomes	(N)	Follow-up	p value
Table 10.1 Effectiveness of physiotherapy techniques (1+) – *continued*			
Conventional physiotherapy techniques			
Alexander technique[370]			
SPDDS 'at best'	88	Post-intervention vs controls	0.04
SPDDS 'at worst'		Post-intervention vs controls	0.01
		6 months vs controls	0.04
		6 months vs controls	0.01
BDI scores		Post-intervention vs controls	0.03
		6 months vs controls	NS
Attitudes to Self Scale		Post-intervention vs controls	NS
		6 months vs controls	0.04

The references cited in this table refer to individual papers within the Cochrane review.[368]

With respect to medication changes:[370]

- The rate of medication change was statistically in favour of Alexander Technique treatment compared with control (p=0.001).
- Fewer participants in the Alexander Technique group changed their medication and yet were not experiencing worsening symptoms (p=0.047). **(1+)**

10.3.3 From evidence to recommendation

There is encouraging RCT evidence of the effectiveness of some of the physiotherapy interventions for people with PD. However, further definitive trials are required to confirm these findings. Additional work is necessary to define what physical therapy interventions are effective in the different stages of the disease. The GDG acknowledge that physiotherapists would not use many of the outcome measures reported in the trial evidence (see Table 10.1). The GDG agree that there is a need for quality-of-life evaluation rated by the patient.

In addition to this evidence, the experience of the GDG members supports the use of physiotherapy interventions in people with PD.

RECOMMENDATIONS

R78   Physiotherapy should be available for people with PD. Particular consideration should
be given to: B
- gait re-education, improvement of balance and flexibility
- enhancement of aerobic capacity
- improvement of movement initiation
- improvement of functional independence, including mobility and activities of daily living
- provision of advice regarding safety in the home environment.

R79 The Alexander Technique may be offered to benefit people with PD by helping them to make lifestyle adjustments that affect both the physical nature of the condition and the person's attitudes to having PD.   C

10.4 Occupational therapy

Occupational therapy (OT) is a profession concerned with promoting health and well-being through occupation. The primary goal of OT is to enable people to participate in the activities of everyday life. Occupational therapists achieve this outcome by enabling people to do things that will enhance their ability to participate or by modifying their environment to better support participation.[375]

Occupational therapists have expertise in assisting people who have disabilities to manage the practical aspects of everyday life. Referral to an occupational therapist can enable people with PD to maximise their current abilities, retain independence for as long as possible and develop their own coping strategies to deal with future problems.[376]

The principles of OT are:

- early intervention to establish rapport, prevent activities and roles being restricted or lost and, where needed, develop appropriate coping strategies
- client-centred assessment and intervention
- development of goals in collaboration with the individual and carer with regular review
- employment of a wide range of interventions to address physical and psychosocial problems to enhance participation in everyday activities such as self-care, mobility, domestic and family roles, work and leisure.

Current UK practice emphasises functional goals centred around independence, safety and confidence, including activities such as transfers, mobility and self-care.[377]

A wide variety of interventions are used in PD. Owing to the individualised nature of the therapeutic process, these may include practising skills, cognitive and sensory cueing strategies, problem solving, advice, education, provision of equipment and environmental adaptations.[378]

What is the effectiveness of occupational therapy versus standard medical therapy in the management of PD?

10.4.1 Methodology

A Cochrane review[379] was found on the effectiveness of OT versus placebo (or no interventions) in people with PD. The review included two randomised, parallel group trials, with a total of 84 people (N=64[380] and N=20[381]).

There were significant differences between the methodologies of the two studies. One trial[380] conducted 20 hours of treatment over 5 weeks with 1-year follow-up while the other trial[381] conducted 12 hours of treatment over 1 month with no follow-up. The methodological limitations of these studies are covered in section 10.3.

Due to the lack of RCT evidence, papers with lower-level study designs (eg non-randomised and/or uncontrolled trials) were also included in the search, but no further papers were found which addressed the effectiveness of OT in the treatment of people with PD.

10.4.2 Evidence statements

With respect to clinical outcome measures:[380]

- Barthel Index score, an assessment of ADL, was maintained over 1 year in those treated with occupational therapy.
- The group without the OT intervention lost an average of 4.6 points (out of a total score of 100) (p values not available).
- The other study[381] reported small differences in mean changes between groups on all outcome measures (motor impairment, activities of daily living, and quality-of-life measures) (p values not available).

10.4.3 From evidence to recommendation

In view of the methodological flaws in the trials and the small numbers of randomised participants, and only one outcome measure reported from one trial, there is insufficient evidence to support the efficacy of OT interventions in PD. However, the GDG support the value of many of the aspects of this therapy, particularly with respect to the provision of aids and adaptations to maintain functional independence in people with PD. There is evidence to support this from one trial where there was maintenance of ADL scores in the treated group but a decline in those not treated. Further trials are required to evaluate the role of different aspects of OT.

Despite this lack of evidence, the experience of the GDG members supports the use of OT interventions in people with PD. It is recognised that, in practice, some of these interventions may be carried out by health professionals other than occupational therapists.

RECOMMENDATION

R80   Occupational therapy should be available for people with PD. Particular consideration
should be given to: D (GPP)
- maintenance of work and family roles, home care and leisure activities
- improvement and maintenance of transfers and mobility
- improvement of personal self-care activities such as eating, drinking, washing and dressing
- environmental issues to improve safety and motor function
- cognitive assessment and appropriate intervention.

10.5 Speech and language therapy

Deterioration in speech is a common manifestation of PD that increases in frequency and intensity with the progress of the disease.

The specific dysarthria resulting from PD is known as hypokinetic dysarthria and it is characterised by:
- monotony with reduced loudness and pitch range
- difficulties in initiating speech
- variable rate

- short rushes of speech
- imprecise consonant
- breathy or harsh voice.

Treatment programmes have focused on specific components of the dysarthria such as respiratory exercise[382] and prosodic exercises.[383] These treatments can be used with individuals or in groups.[384]

Lee Silverman Voice Treatment (LSVT) is a speech therapy programme developed specifically for individuals with PD. It focuses on improving voice loudness with immediate carry over into daily communication. The intensive nature of the programme helps individuals with PD to recognise that their voice is too soft, convince them that a louder voice is within normal limits and makes them comfortable using the new louder voice. It is now provided by certified clinicians in England.

Some people with PD may benefit from use of augmentative and alternative communication devices, which can include the use of:
- alphabet boards
- pacing boards
- voice amplifiers
- digitised speech output systems
- recorded voice messages
- delayed auditory feedback[385]
- microcomputer-based wearable biofeedback device.[386]

What is the effectiveness of speech and language therapy versus standard medical therapy or control in the treatment of speech disturbance in PD?

10.5.1 Methodology

A systematic review[387] was found which addressed the efficacy of speech and language therapy versus standard medical therapy in people with PD.

The review included three RCTs,[384,388,389] with a total sample size of 63. One of these trials used the LSVT technique,[389] whereas the rest used the more conventional speech and language therapy techniques. No raw numerical data were available from one of these studies,[384] so data on only 41 participants were available from the review's[387] analysis. Another included study[388] showed the intervention groups differed significantly from one another at baseline on a number of outcome measures, but no further analysis was provided.

There were significant differences in the intensity of the speech and language therapy intervention between studies. One trial[388] treated participants for 10 hours over 4 weeks, another trial[389] provided treatment for 16 hours over 4 weeks and a third trial[384] treated people for 35–40 hours over 2 weeks.

10.5.2 Evidence statements

With respect to the assessment of speech impairment:
- One study[388] found total impairment with the Frenchay Dysarthria Assessment improved in the intervention group compared with the placebo (p<0.05), showing an overall

improvement in the dysarthria score, while all participants in the untreated group showed lower scores with a significant deterioration (p<0.05).

- Another study[384] reported that the scores of the Dysarthria Profile were comparable at baseline, but immediately after therapy the scores were significantly higher in the treatment group (p<0.05).

With respect to vocal loudness:

- In two trials objective loudness improved by 11 dB[388] and by 5.4 dB[389] (p<0.005) immediately after therapy.
- This gain was reduced by 3.5 dB[389] after 6 months but was still significantly in favour of therapy (p<0.05).[389]
- Mean objective loudness of speech when the participants were asked to describe a picture improved by 5.2 dB (p<0.025) and this improvement was maintained over 6 months (4.2 dB, p<0.02).[389]
- The reading loudness of participants receiving LSVT was more than the placebo group immediately after therapy (p<0.001) and improvement was mostly maintained (p<0.005) at 6 months.[389]
- Mean objective loudness improved when people were asked to give a prolonged 'a' (12.1 dB, p<0.001) and this was mostly maintained (9.4 dB, p<0.001) at 6 months.[389]
- Maximum vocal loudness increased after therapy[388] by 16 dB (p<0.01).
- Mean pitch range increased in the therapy group by 66 Hz (162.7 to 228.3) and remained virtually static in the placebo group.[388]

10.5.3 From evidence to recommendation

Although there is good preliminary evidence of the efficacy of speech and language therapy for speech disorders in PD, this is based on data from only 41 people with maximum follow-up of only 12 weeks. Much of the positive data concerns the unique North American therapy LSVT. While some therapists in England and Wales have attended the mandatory training programme for this intervention, it is not widely available at present. The GDG was also concerned about the practicalities of 16 1-hour treatment sessions in the context of the NHS financial climate.

There is little evidence comparing speech and language therapy to standard medical therapy or control. The GDG were aware of a body of evidence that addresses use of LSVT compared with other speech and language therapy techniques.[390–393] In addition to this, the experience of the GDG members supports the use of speech and language therapy intervention in people with PD.

In the section on dysphagia (Chapter 9) the potential contribution that could be made by speech and language therapist interventions is discussed.

RECOMMENDATION

R81   Speech and language therapy should be available for people with PD. Particular consideration should be given to:

- improvement of vocal loudness and pitch range, including speech therapy programmes such as LSVT   **B**
- teaching strategies to optimise speech intelligibility   **D (GPP)**
- ensuring an effective means of communication is maintained throughout the course of the disease, including use of assistive technologies   **D (GPP)**
- review and management to support the safety and efficiency of swallowing and to minimise the risk of aspiration.   **D (GPP)**

11 | Palliative care in Parkinson's disease

11.1 Introduction

In the absence of any curative treatment, the management of PD remains largely palliative despite the huge advances that have been made in medical knowledge. The principles of palliative care should be applied throughout the course of the disease and not limited to the terminal end-of-life period.

Palliative care can be defined in the following way:

> *The active total care of patients whose disease is not responsive to curative treatment. Control of pain and other symptoms and of psychological, social and spiritual problems is paramount.*

The goal of palliative care is achievement of the best quality of life for patients and their families.[394]

Palliative care is an approach that improves the quality of life of patients and their families facing the problems associated with life-threatening illness. It does not necessarily mean the use of specialist care services but should focus on prevention and relief of suffering with early identification, impeccable assessment, and treatment of pain and other physical, psychological and spiritual problems.

The issues common to malignant and non-malignant conditions, that are the focus of palliative care, can be categorised[395] as:

- physical: pain, breathlessness, anorexia, immobility and constipation
- social: loss of employment, role change, fear for dependants
- psychological: depression, fear and anxiety, uncertainty, guilt
- existential: religious, non-religious, meaning of life, why?

11.2 The palliative phase of Parkinson's disease

The needs of patients in the palliative care stage of PD are not always identified or satisfied.[396] Over time, progression of the underlying disease process makes interventions less effective and they may be associated with intercurrent illnesses. As a result, patients become increasingly disabled and dependent. This physical disability is often combined with cognitive dysfunction and depression.

The 'palliative phase' in PD has been defined by:[397]

- inability to tolerate adequate dopaminergic therapy
- unsuitability for surgery
- the presence of advanced comorbidity.

The duration of time spent in each of the stages of PD is variable. From an audit of 73 patients undertaken in Cornwall[398] the mean duration of disease was 14.6 years. The time spent in the four stages was: diagnosis 1.5 years; maintenance 6 years; complex 5 years, and palliative care

2.2 years. This reinforces the view that 'palliative care' in PD does not equate with imminent end of life, but that the emphasis of care will shift from a 'therapeutic' pharmacological approach to one that places greater emphasis on quality of life issues. This is in recognition of the shortened remaining lifespan of the patient and the inadequacy of current medications to meet the increase in needs.

The care of people with PD is best undertaken in a multidisciplinary way throughout each stage of the disease. The palliative care approach should be utilised by all health professionals throughout these stages. It should also be possible to seek advice from specialist palliative care teams, not just at the end of life, but at any stage after diagnosis with the main aims of care to provide symptom relief, prevent complications, minimise distress, maintain patient dignity and provide counselling. With more complex difficulties, the specialist palliative care team may, on agreement, become temporarily or regularly involved with input for the patient or their family, and in supporting the usual professional carers.

The NSF for Long-term (Neurological) Conditions (2005)[14] focuses on the palliative care needs of patients with chronic disabling conditions such as PD in 'Quality requirement 9: palliative care'.

11.2.1 Palliative care and carers

Management of the palliative stage must always be in the context of the patient and the family/caregiver. Recognising the needs of carers of people with PD at an early stage will help enable patients to be maintained at home for as long as possible. Many will have been in the role of carer for a significant number of years and have become 'experts' in PD themselves. Realistic goals need to be agreed jointly by the patient/family and the multidisciplinary team caring for the patient. Respite periods, both for short and longer periods and to meet planned and emergency needs, are particularly important. The White Paper 'Your health, your care, your say' highlights the need for carer support. It may also be useful to refer to a carer care pathway to recognise some of the problems carers may experience. When looking at specific information and support for carers, the PDS provides useful information sheets for carers.[399,400]

11.2.2 Care homes

While the majority of people with PD will cope at home for many years, increasing dependency in the palliative stage, when the care needs exceed the ability of their family or community to cope, will frequently lead to admission into care home settings. This may be due to increased disability or the result of a combination of disability and social factors when the burden of caring becomes too great. In particular, PD studies suggest[401,402] that care home admission is often provoked by hallucinations. Admission of patients into care homes carries with it a greater mortality.[401,402] These trials found that all PD patients admitted into care homes died within 2 years of admission. PD may affect 5–10% of nursing home residents.[403] Guidance on caring for people in care homes in the palliative stage is available.[404–406]

11.2.3 Social costs

Social services will play an increasingly greater role in palliative care stages; in particular to address issues that may arise from increased disability and dependency. Results from a study[10] looking into the economic impact of PD showed that:

- Total social services costs accounted for 34% of total costs and tended to increase with increasing age.
- Total NHS costs accounted for 38% of total costs and tended to fall with increasing age.
- Total annual direct costs were £4,189 for patients living at home; £15,355 for patients whose time was divided between home and an institution; and £19,338 for patients in full-time institutional care.

Wherever the patient resides, their condition should be monitored to ensure comfort and quality of life is maintained. However it may be difficult to assess their needs in a hospital outpatient environment. Day hospital attendance may be easier or a PDNS or other key worker may visit at home. Visiting in the home environment is less stressful for the patient, carer and care staff, and allows time for more detailed discussion, advice, education and counselling.

11.2.4 Withdrawal of drugs

In later stages of PD there may be the need to withdraw dopaminergic drugs due to lack of drug efficacy and increasing sensitivity to unwanted effects such as hallucinations. As a general guide, medication withdrawal should be managed with help from the specialist clinician and PDNS. Where possible drug withdrawal should be gradual in order to achieve the best balance between relief of symptoms and minimal side effects. Patients and carers at this stage will often agree to reduce medications, exchanging greater levels of physical disability for increased mental clarity. This situation should however be reviewed on an ongoing basis as frequent adjustments may be required to maintain this balance.

11.2.5 Pressure ulcers

Immobility in the palliative care phase of PD places individuals at risk of pressure ulcer development, and an assessment of risk for pressure ulcers should be a priority. Most pressure ulcers occur over a bony prominence, but if contractures of the limbs have developed with immobility and the altered body shape of PD, this may result in pressure sores appearing in more unusual locations.

Carers will require support and education in understanding how to move and handle patients safely. Additional information can be found in:
- NICE documents:
  - Pressure relieving devices guidelines[407]
  - Pressure ulcer risk assessment and prevention guidelines[408]
- Royal College of Nursing documents:
  - Clinical practice guidelines on pressure ulcer risk assessment and prevention: implementation guide and audit protocol.[409]

11.2.6 End-of-life issues

In July 2004 the Department of Health (England) started an initiative so that all adult patients nearing the end of life, irrespective of diagnosis, will have access to high-quality specialist palliative care. The focus was to train and equip healthcare professionals with the knowledge and skills to support patients to live and die in the place of their choice. Three key documents make up the basis of this 'End of Life Initiative':

- Preferred Place of Care Plan[410]
- Gold Standards Framework[411]
- Liverpool Care of the Dying Pathway.[412]

Increasingly, initiatives such as these have resulted in district general hospitals (DGHs), primary care and care homes achieving:

- increased advance care planning
- greater choice for patients in where they wish to live and die
- decreased emergency admissions of patients who wish to die at home
- decreased number of older people transferred from a care home to a DGH in the last week of life.

What are the end-of-life palliative care needs of PD patients and what treatments are available? These aspects are currently being explored within the neurological conditions policy group of the National Council for Palliative Care, working closely with the PDS. www.ncpc.org.uk/policy_unit/neuro_pg.html

11.2.7 Methodology

No trials were found which addressed end-of-life palliative care needs of PD patients and what treatments are available.

11.2.8 From evidence to recommendation

The needs of patients in the palliative care stage of PD are often under-recognised and considered too late in their care. Better understanding of the complexity of the manifestations of the disease, its innate variability, and the roles of the extended team members, which may or may not include the palliative care team, can help to improve care and reduce distress. Care needs to be supported by good care planning since many problems can be predicted or avoided with appropriate strategies.

RECOMMENDATIONS

R82   Palliative care requirements of people with PD should be considered throughout all phases of the disease.   **D (GPP)**

R83   People with PD and their carers should be given the opportunity to discuss end-of-life issues with appropriate healthcare professionals.   **D (GPP)**

11.3 Ethical issues

Patients and their families need to be allowed to have time to come to terms with the fact that the disease has reached a stage where no more can be done. Decisions may need to be made about management and treatment in the future, and end-of-life decisions (ie do-not-resuscitate policies and advance directives (living wills)). These are never easy issues to discuss but they can provide an opportunity for the person with PD to state treatment preferences should they lose their capacity for decision making in the future. They derive their authority from the principle of informed consent and the promotion of personal autonomy and should be considered before mental or physical disability precludes their completion.

Additional information that may be of help includes the British Geriatrics Society Compendium advance directives section (**www.bgs.org.uk**), and the BMA (**www.bma.org.uk**).

12 | Research recommendations

12.1 Future research recommendations

The questions below are not in order of priority.

▷ Question 1: Do any of the agents with preclinical neuroprotective properties in PD models have any clinically worthwhile protective effects in PD?

Population	People with early PD: some trials with patients on no medication; other trials may randomise patients stabilised on symptomatic medication Any gender, age, ethnic group Trials performed in secondary care.
Intervention	Systematic reviews in the USA have identified 12 agents that require study (Table 6.2). The UK could contribute to the raft of ongoing studies that are funded by the National Institute for Neurologic Disorders and Stroke (NINDS) and the Michael J Fox Foundation Support should also be given to innovative surgical approaches to neuroprotection
Comparison	Each putative neuroprotectant versus placebo in double-blind parallel design or delayed-start design trial
Outcome	Total UPDRS change

Table 6.2 NINDS selected candidate neuroprotective drugs in Parkinson's disease[100]
Caffeine
Co-enzyme Q_{10}*
Creatine*
GM-1 ganglioside
GPI-1485*
Minocycline*
Nicotine
Oestrogen
MAOB inhibitors (rasagiline§ and selegiline)
Dopamine agonists (ropinirole§ and pramipexole§)

*In phase II or III studies in North America.
§Further neuroprotection trials may be performed by manufacturer.

Explanatory paragraph

At present there is no agent that slows the progression of PD. Patients want such a 'cure' for their condition. The NHS requires neuroprotectants to reduce the burden of disability caused by PD, thereby reducing the direct and indirect costs of caring for an increasing number of people with the condition.

While the pharmaceutical industry is trying to develop new putative neuroprotectants, 12 existing agents have been identified which may slow PD progression (Table 6.2). A systematic trial programme examining these agents is ongoing in the USA (Net-PD) funded by the NINDS and the Michael J Fox Foundation. Agents are being screened in small 'futility studies' using historical control data for decline in total UPDRS scores. Agents that delay progression by more than 30% will go through to larger definitive studies.

The first futility study showed that both minocycline and GPI-1485 significantly delay decline in total UPDRS by more than 30%. However, a small placebo comparator group also showed a similar effect, raising doubts about the use of historical controls.

Future Net-PD trials may use patients already established on symptomatic therapies. There are many more such patients than those who are untreated thereby allowing future neuroprotection trials to be much larger.

The recent rasagiline delayed-start design trial versus placebo (see section 6.5) raised the possibility that this may be a useful trial design to examine neuroprotection. Further pharmaceutical industry trials using this design are planned. This would be another option for UK neuroprotection trials.

UK investigators have recently carried out neurorestoration trials with intra-putaminal infusion of GDNF, although these have now been stopped. Support for further surgical approaches to neuroprotection in PD should be considered.

▷ Question 2: Which people with PDD benefit from cholinesterase inhibitor drugs and/or memantine, and is the use of these agents cost-effective?

Population	Patients with PD of more than 2 years' duration (to exclude dementia with Lewy bodies patients) and dementia defined according to DSM-IV criteria or new MDS Task Force criteria for PDD (due mid-2006) Patients stratified according to pattern and severity of cognitive impairment and neuropsychiatric burden (eg visual hallucinations) Concomitant use of stable atypical antipsychotic regimen will be permitted Any sex, age, ethnic group Trials performed in secondary care
Intervention	Donepezil/rivastigmine/galantamine/memantine
Comparison	Cholinesterase inhibitor/memantine versus placebo in RCT design
Outcome	Change in cognition according to validated scales (eg ADAS-cog, new MDS Task Force instrument for PDD – due mid-2006) Neuropsychiatric Inventory Caregiver stress scales Health economics using disease-specific models

Explanatory paragraph

A recent systematic review indicates that 24–31% of PD patients have dementia, and that 3–4% of the dementia in the general population is due to PDD. The estimated prevalence of PDD in the general population aged 65 years and older is 0.2–0.5%. PDD is associated with increased mortality, caregiver stress and nursing home admission.

A large RCT of rivastigmine in PDD showed improvements in primary and secondary end-points but the clinical significance of these benefits is uncertain. It is likely that the modest mean improvements reflect heterogeneity of response, with some patients responding far better than others; this is supported by expert opinion via open-label prescribing. In addition, health economic analysis has not been performed in trials of cholinesterase inhibitors in PDD using disease-specific models.

Identifying responsive subgroups of patients with PDD with demonstrable cost-effectiveness would focus effective targeting of cholinesterase inhibitors and/or memantine. The process of identifying these patients would also lead to the development of protocols for prescribing and assessment, together with robust guidelines regarding whether drug usage is maintained or discontinued.

▷ Question 3: Is treating mild to moderate depression in PD with an antidepressant cost-effective?

Population	People with any stage of PD with mild to moderate depression according to a depression rating scale. Patients with severe depression will be excluded, as treatment is mandatory Any sex, age, ethnic group Trials performed in secondary care
Intervention	Any SSRI class of antidepressant
Comparison	SSRI antidepressant versus no treatment in a pragmatic open-label design
Outcomes	Quality of life rated by disease specific (PDQ-39) and generic (SF-36, EuroQol) measures Health economics Depression scores on accepted depression rating scale

Explanatory paragraph

Cross-sectional studies have shown that depression affects around 40% of patients with PD and has a major impact on quality of life. In most cases depression is mild to moderate in severity and is often missed by the clinician caring for the patient.

The GDG recommends a study that would screen secondary care PD clinic populations for mild to moderate depression. Participants would then be treated with any SSRI class antidepressant or no such treatment in an open-label fashion. This would be a large-scale pragmatic trial.

If screening for and treating mild to moderate depression is cost-effective, this will add to the evidence base for the management of depression in PD and may have considerable impact on the next update of this guideline.

▷ Question 4: Are supportive therapies in PD cost-effective?
(a) Is physiotherapy in PD cost-effective?

Population	People with any stage of PD Any sex, age, ethnic group Trials based in secondary care with primary care support
Intervention	Best practice NHS physiotherapy
Comparison	Pragmatic parallel design trial comparing no treatment with physiotherapy
Outcome	Quality of life rated by disease-specific (PDQ-39) and generic (SF-36, EuroQol) measures Health economics Disease-specific and therapy-specific outcomes including: gait, balance, posture, transfers, and reaching and grasping

Explanatory paragraph

The evidence to support the use of physiotherapy in PD is limited and yet patients feel that it is effective. Many patients are referred for such therapy in the NHS with little idea of its value or whether it has any long-term benefits. In contrast, many other patients cannot access such therapy due to limited provision of service.

The GDG recommends a pragmatic trial performed in units that already have access to physiotherapy services. This is likely to be in the elderly care setting because neurologists have limited access to such treatments. An NHS subvention will be required to ensure adequate therapy resources are available for the trial.

Many prevalent cases of PD will have already received such therapies, so the trial will recruit incident cases. This will require a long recruitment period, a large number of centres or both.

A large trial of cueing therapy (The Rescue Project) in PD has recently been completed but is yet to report.[413] The data from this can act as pilot material for the new trial.

If physiotherapy is cost-effective, the provision of service needs to be increased. If it is not cost-effective, services can be diverted to other conditions.

Future trials will then need to examine which components of physiotherapy are effective and whether it is effective in the earlier stages of the disease.

▷   (b) Is OT in PD cost-effective?

Population	People with any stage of PD Any sex, age, ethnic group Trials based in secondary care with primary care support
Intervention	Best practice NHS occupational therapy
Comparison	Pragmatic parallel design trial comparing no treatment with OT
Outcome	Quality of life rated by disease-specific (PDQ-39) and generic (SF-36, EuroQol) measures Health economics Secondary outcomes to include disease-specific and therapy-specific measures

Explanatory paragraph

The evidence to support the use of OT in PD is limited and yet patients feel it is effective. Many patients are referred for such therapy in the NHS with little idea of its value or whether it has any long-term benefits. In contrast, many other patients cannot access such therapy due to limited provision of service.

The GDG recommends a pragmatic trial performed in units that already have access to occupational therapy services. This is likely to be in the elderly care setting because neurologists have poor access to such treatments. An NHS subvention will be required to ensure adequate therapy resources are available for the trial.

Many prevalent cases of PD will have already received such therapies, so the trial will recruit incident cases. This will require a long recruitment period, a large number of centres or both.

A pilot study of OT in PD is underway in Birmingham. This will provide invaluable data upon which to plan the substantive trial.

If OT is cost-effective, the provision of service needs to be increased. If it is not cost-effective, services can be diverted to other conditions.

Future trials will then need to examine what components of OT are effective.

▷ (c) Is NHS speech and language therapy in PD cost-effective?

Population	People with any stage of PD who have developed speech problems as defined by the observing clinician Any sex, age, ethnic group Trials based in secondary care with primary care support
Intervention	Best practice NHS speech and language therapy
Comparison	Pragmatic trial comparing NHS speech and language therapy with no treatment
Outcome	Quality of life rated by disease-specific (PDQ-39) and generic (SF-36, EuroQol) measures Health economics Measures of intelligibility Secondary outcomes to include disease-specific and therapy-specific measures

Explanatory paragraph

The evidence to support the use of speech and language therapy in PD is limited and yet patients feel that it is effective. The provision of this service in the NHS is patchy with some patients not receiving speech and language therapy when it may be appropriate.

The GDG recommends a trial that is preceded by survey work to identify current and best practice speech and language therapy for PD in the UK. Similar work has already been performed for physiotherapy and OT to prepare for analogous trials.

In this pragmatic trial, standard NHS speech and language therapy would be compared with no treatment. While most PD units will have access to some speech and language therapy service, this may be insufficient for trial purposes so an NHS subvention would be required.

It is likely that a pilot study will be required to assess issues concerning availability of services, recruitment rates, etc.

If speech and language therapy is cost-effective, the provision of service needs to be increased. If it is not cost-effective, services can be diverted to other conditions.

Future trials will then need to examine what components of speech and language therapy are effective.

▷ Question 5: Which diagnostic investigations for PD and potential biomarkers of its progression are clinically useful and cost-effective?

Population	People with suspected PD Any sex, age, ethnic group Trials performed in secondary care
Interventions	(1) Development of existing and novel diagnostic tests to differentiate PD from (a) non-parkinsonism (ie normality and essential tremor) and (b) other parkinsonian disorders (ie PSP, MSA, corticobasal degeneration) (2) Development of biomarkers to follow the progression of PD, mainly to be used in neuroprotection trials
Comparison	Diagnostic accuracy of test versus UK PDS Brain Bank Criteria or ^{123}I-FP-CIT SPECT
Outcome	Well-designed diagnostic studies using receiver-operator characteristic curves were appropriate to establish standard diagnostic clinimetrics of investigations (eg sensitivity and specificity).

Explanatory paragraph

The diagnosis of PD remains clinical. ^{123}I-FP-CIT SPECT may be of additional help in a small proportion of clinically uncertain cases. The diagnostic error rate on presentation may be as high as 10% in expert hands, which may lead to inappropriate therapy and distress following revision of the diagnosis.

A systematic approach led by university researchers and funded by the government would expedite the evaluation of existing and new diagnostic techniques.

The considerable debate surrounding biomarkers to measure the progression of PD has highlighted the need for further studies in this area. More work on existing techniques (eg SPECT and PET) is required and the development of new potential markers of progression is urgently required.

12.2 General research recommendations

These general research recommendations are in addition to the prioritised research recommendations covered in the preceding section. These were gaps in the evidence base that were identified by the GDG when reviewing the literature for the guideline. The GDG recognises that there are many areas of ongoing research activity in the diagnosis, treatment and management of PD. The following were agreed as broad areas for future research development.

Methodology

There were methodological limitations in many of the studies reviewed in the guideline. The GDG agreed that there was a need to make some general recommendations on the design of future research trials in PD.

The following issues should be considered in future trial design:

- Sample size calculations should be performed before the study to ensure large enough numbers of patients are included to prevent false-negative conclusions.
- UK Brain Bank diagnostic criteria should be used to ensure all trial participants have idiopathic PD.
- Trials should attempt to include a more representative spectrum of patients with PD, particularly the elderly and those with comorbidity.
- Outcome measures should include patient-rated quality-of-life instruments and health economics evaluations.
- Patients should be followed for prolonged periods.
- An intention-to-treat analysis of the data from all randomised participants should be performed.
- All reporting of results should be to CONSORT standards.[414]

Diagnosis

In the development of diagnostic tests for PD in the future, study designs should be improved to include, for example:

- blinding of investigators
- assessment of established cases then assessment of newly diagnosed cases with prospective follow-up
- reporting of appropriate statistics (including sensitivity, specificity, positive and negative predictive values).

More research is needed in the use of MRI, magnetic resonance volumetry, MRS, PET, MIBZ-SPECT, IBZM-SPECT, transcranial ultrasound and smell testing as diagnostic tools to accurately differentiate PD from controls, those with essential tremor and those with other parkinsonian conditions before further conclusions can be reached regarding their value.

Many of these investigations are expensive with limited availability. It would be particularly useful to develop inexpensive tests for PD based on serum or cerebrospinal fluid biomarkers or more sophisticated bedside tests; for example, olfaction, eye movements, neuropsychological testing and detailed movement analysis.

Studies should be done to examine the possibility of combining two or more diagnostic tests to improve accuracy. This is particularly applicable to less expensive investigations. In addition, studies should also compare promising diagnostic tests directly (eg SPECT scanning with objective smell identification).

Neuroprotection

Careful consideration must be given to the design of neuroprotection trials in PD in the future to avoid the mistakes of the past.

A systematic approach to the development of neuroprotection trials in PD should be adopted in England and Wales along the lines of, and possibly in collaboration with, the NINDS in the USA. From a societal perspective, it would be more cost-effective to slow or halt the progression of PD than to continue to treat it symptomatically.

The UK has recently led neurorestoration trials using intra-putaminal GDNF infusions in PD. Support for similar trials in the future will be imperative.

Methods to improve neuroprotection trial design include:

- Washout of drug at the end of the trial should be prolonged or trial should be done in patients not requiring symptomatic medication (ie very early disease)
- Future longitudinal clinicopathological studies are required to evaluate the ultimate diagnosis and prognosis of patients bearing an initial clinical diagnosis of PD who are found to have normal SPECT and/or PET images.
- Misdiagnosis must be taken into account when sample size calculations are performed.
- Larger and longer studies may be able to show more clinically meaningful effects.
- Standardisation of imaging methodology with blind evaluation of results should be better.
- There should be repeated imaging after dose titration and after drug withdrawal at end of trial.
- If the predicted therapeutic effect is mild or slight, trials need to be much larger (ie thousands of patients).
- Large explanatory trials in early disease should be rolled on into pragmatic long-term trials reflecting real-life practice with quality-of-life and health economics outcomes.

Symptomatic therapy

Future clinical trials examining the effectiveness of symptomatic therapies in PD should be longer and larger than those in the past to provide more reliable evidence of the long-term effects of treatments. Such trials should use robust clinical criteria for the diagnosis of PD. Results should be reported on an intention-to-treat basis using CONSORT reporting guidelines. Crossover trials should report the results of the first half of the study separately from the overall results and should have a sufficiently long washout period to prevent carry-over effects.

More data on the comparative efficacy and safety of the most commonly used symptomatic therapies for early PD are required. In particular, we need more information on the relative merits of levodopa, dopamine agonists, amantadine, anticholinergics and MAOB inhibitors in terms of quality-of-life and health economics outcomes.

Clinicians require more data on the comparative efficacy and safety of adjuvant therapies for later PD once levodopa has been commenced and motor complications have developed. There is insufficient information on which to base a decision whether to add a dopamine agonist, a COMT inhibitor or an MAOB inhibitor.

The PD MED trial is comparing levodopa, dopamine agonists and MAOB inhibitors in early PD and adjuvant therapy in later PD with dopamine agonists, COMT inhibitors and MAOB inhibitors using quality-of-life and health economics outcomes.

Non-motor features

Depression is common in PD, but further work is required to:

- develop suitable ways to screen for mild depression in clinic populations
- obtain information on the value of cognitive behavioural therapy
- obtain more trial data on the efficacy and safety of SSRIs and other modern classes of antidepressant in PD.

Further work is needed to evaluate the role of electroconvulsive therapy in drug and cognitive behavioural therapy-refractory depression.

Additional trials should be performed with memory-enhancing agents in PDD. Trials are needed to compare the effects of atypical antipsychotics with those of memory-enhancing agents in PDD.

Further research is required to evaluate treatments for daytime hypersomnolence, constipation, bladder disturbance, autonomic dysfunction, and RBD associated with PD.

Other key interventions

In the development of evidence to support physiotherapy intervention, future research should include large, well-designed trials to investigate:
- the optimal stage in the condition for referral to a physiotherapy practitioner
- the benefit of exercise for people in the different stages of the condition in relation to maintenance of their movement capability and function
- the role of optimising physical capacity to delay the onset and manifestation of disability
- the benefit of physiotherapy in preventing falls in people with PD
- the benefit of physiotherapy in maintaining confidence to move in people with PD
- the benefit of multi- and interdisciplinary intervention (including physiotherapy) in enabling a good quality of life in people with PD and their family and carers
- physiotherapy as an adjunct to change in medical and surgical intervention.

Further large, well-designed trials are required to evaluate the impact of occupational therapy for people with PD, including large, well-designed trials to investigate:
- the optimal stage for referral to OT
- the benefit of OT in maintaining or optimising safety and independence in transfers, mobility and personal care, and in reducing risk/ frequency of falls
- the benefit of OT in maintaining or optimising work, family, leisure and recreational roles and activities, according to the specific wishes and needs of the individual with PD
- the value of OT in the management of anxiety and depression
- the benefit of provision of information and advice about assistive aids, equipment and wheelchairs, and about practical and financial support and services
- the benefit of OT in improvement of hand function, including handwriting/management of micrographia
- the value of education and advice about the self-management of symptoms, especially where these are experienced in 'a pre-drug management phase', where symptoms are drug resistant or where drug side effects limit their use
- the value of a multi-interdisciplinary intervention (including OT) in enabling a good quality of life in people with PD, their families and carers.

Further research is required into the impact of speech and language therapy intervention for people with PD, including large, well-designed trials to investigate:

- different therapy programmes and their impact on features such as vocal loudness and overall communication competency/intelligibility
- treatment for dysphagia
- trials of different intensities of treatments and their impact on communication over time
- the optimal timing for intervention
- the benefit of using assistive augmentative communication devices for people with PD
- the benefit of speech and language therapy intervention on quality of life, such as feelings of social isolation
- the impact of communication difficulties on family and carers and whether this can be reduced with intervention.

APPENDICES

Appendix A: The scope of the guideline

Guideline title

Parkinson's disease: diagnosis, management and treatment of Parkinson's disease in primary and secondary care

Background

The National Institute for Health and Clinical Excellence (NICE or 'the Institute') has commissioned the National Collaborating Centre for Chronic Conditions to develop a clinical guideline on Parkinson's disease (PD) for use in the NHS in England and Wales. This follows referral of the topic by the Department of Health and Welsh Assembly Government (see below). The guideline will provide recommendations for good practice that are based on the best available evidence of clinical and cost-effectiveness.

The Institute's clinical guidelines will support the implementation of national service frameworks (NSFs) in those aspects of care where a framework has been published. The statements in each NSF reflect the evidence that was used at the time the framework was prepared. The clinical guidelines and technology appraisals published by the Institute after an NSF has been issued will have the effect of updating the framework.

Clinical need for the guideline

Parkinson's disease is a progressive neurodegenerative condition leading to death of the dopamine-containing cells of the substantia nigra. The 'cardinal signs' of the disease are rest tremor, rigidity, and hypokinesia. Postural instability and falls occur later during the course of the condition. Additional common findings are asymmetric onset of symptoms and symptomatic response to L-dopa (levodopa). Although predominantly a movement disorder, cognitive impairments including dementia do occur. All of these problems lead to significant disability and handicap with impaired quality of life for both patients and their carers and increased healthcare costs.

Parkinson's disease is one of the commonest neurological conditions. It is estimated to affect up to 160 per 100,000 of the general population with an annual incidence of 15–20 per 100,000. Many population studies have shown the rising prevalence with age (up to 2% of the population aged 80 and over). Around 1 in 7 cases are diagnosed below the age of 60 years.

The costs of treatment have been estimated at between £560,000 and £1.6 million per 100,000 of the population. Significant cost drivers include the onset of motor fluctuations, psychiatric symptoms, and institutional care. Parkinson's disease is a frequent cause of falls, fractures, and hospital admission and is therefore a costly disease, especially in the later stages.[10,362,415]

The guideline

The guideline development process is described in detail in three booklets that are available from the NICE website (see 'Further information'). *The guideline development process: information for stakeholders*[13] describes how organisations can become involved in the development of a guideline.

This document is the scope. It defines exactly what this guideline will (and will not) examine, and what the guideline developers will consider. The scope is based on the referral from the Department of Health and Welsh Assembly Government (see below).

The areas that will be addressed by the guideline are described in the following sections.

Population

Groups that will be covered:
- both sexes over 20 years of age
- diagnoses: Parkinson's disease and parkinsonism
- treatment: idiopathic Parkinson's disease only.

Groups that will not be covered:
- juvenile onset Parkinson's disease (<20 years)
- pregnant females
- treatment: parkinsonism (a neurological disorder that manifests with hypokinesia, tremor, or muscular rigidity) and other tremulous disorders (eg essential tremor) – except for accurate differential diagnosis.

Healthcare setting

The guideline will cover the care received from primary, secondary and tertiary NHS care settings.

Clinical management

The guideline will cover the following aspects of management.

Diagnosis and monitoring:
- clinical expert diagnosis (using UK PDS Brain Bank Criteria)
    - versus non-expert diagnosis
    - versus post-mortem gold standard
- other diagnostic tests (eg acute levodopa and apomorphine tests, radionuclide imaging: PET and SPECT, magnetic resonance imaging, magnetic resonance volumetry, magnetic resonance spectroscopy, growth hormone stimulation test).

Communication and education:
- communication of the diagnosis and patient understanding
- patient education (self-help), both specific and generic issues, including falls prevention

Pharmacotherapy:
- prevention of progression – the use of neuro-protective therapy (eg dopamine agonists, MAOB inhibitors, amantadine, co-enzyme Q_{10}, vitamins).
- functional disability – treatment of early disease with:
    - immediate-release levodopa
    - modified-release levodopa

- – dopamine agonists
- – MAOB inhibitors
- – amantadine
- – anticholinergics
- – beta-blockers.

- adjuvant pharmacotherapy:
  - – dopamine agonists
  - – COMT inhibitors
  - – MAOB inhibitors
  - – amantadine
  - – intermittent apomorphine injections and continuous infusion
  - – treatment of non-motor symptoms (eg sleep disturbance).

Non-pharmacological management:
- current surgical options (eg deep brain stimulation)
- physiotherapy
- speech and language therapy
- occupational therapy
- Parkinson's disease nurse specialists

Neuropsychiatric conditions
- psychosis management specific to PD
- depression management specific to PD
- dementia management specific to PD.

Palliative care:
- end-of-life issues specific to PD.

The guideline will not cover the following aspects of intervention/management.
- radical therapies that do not form common clinical management: fetal cell transplantation; stem cells; genes that code protein responsible for producing dopamine; drugs that block the action of glutamate; GDNF; viral transfection
- comorbidities in Parkinson's disease (except where treatment will differ from treatment of these comorbidities in patients without Parkinson's disease)
- generic health problems where the care for people with Parkinson's disease does not differ to that of the general population (eg constipation).

Audit support within guideline

The guideline will include Level 1 clinical audit criteria.

Referral from the Department of Health and Welsh Assembly Government

The Department of Health and the Welsh Assembly Government asked the Institute in May 2002:

'To prepare clinical guidelines for the NHS in England and Wales for the diagnosis, management and treatment of Parkinson's disease in both primary and secondary care settings, including examination of the evidence for the effectiveness of management of the condition by physiotherapy, speech, language and occupational therapies, self-help, drug therapies and surgery.'

Appendix B: Details of questions and literature searches

	Table B1 Details of questions and literature searches		
Question ID	**Question wording**	**Study type filters used**	**Database and year**
DIAG1	How effective is clinical expert diagnosis (using UK PDS Brain Bank Criteria) vs non-expert diagnosis in diagnosing patients with Parkinson's disease?	Diagnosis	Medline 1966–2005 Embase 1980–2005 Cochrane 1800–2005 CINAHL 1982–2005
DIAG2	How effective is clinical expert diagnosis (using UK PDS Brain Bank Criteria) vs the post-mortem gold standard in diagnosing patients with Parkinson's disease?	Diagnosis	Medline 1966–2005 Embase 1980–2005 Cochrane 1800–2005 CINAHL 1982–2005
DIAG3	How effective is acute levodopa testing and apomorphine testing vs long-term clinical follow-up in determining an accurate diagnosis in patients with a parkinsonian syndrome?	Diagnosis	Medline 1966–2005 Embase 1980–2005 Cochrane 1800–2005 CINAHL 1982–2005
DIAG4a	How effective is magnetic resonance imaging vs long-term clinical follow-up in determining an accurate diagnosis in patients with a parkinsonian syndrome?	Diagnosis	Medline 1966–2005 Embase 1980–2005 Cochrane 1800–2005 CINAHL 1982–2005
DIAG4b	How effective is magnetic resonance volumetry vs long-term clinical follow-up in determining an accurate diagnosis in patients with a parkinsonian syndrome?	Diagnosis	Medline 1966–2005 Embase 1980–2005 Cochrane 1800–2005 CINAHL 1982–2005
DIAG4c	How effective is magnetic resonance spectroscopy vs long-term clinical follow-up in determining an accurate diagnosis in patients with a parkinsonian syndrome?	Diagnosis	Medline 1966–2005 Embase 1980–2005 Cochrane 1800–2005 CINAHL 1982–2005
DIAG6	How effective is positron emission tomography vs long-term clinical follow-up in determining an accurate diagnosis in patients with a parkinsonian syndrome?	Diagnosis	Medline 1966–2005 Embase 1980–2005 Cochrane 1800–2005 CINAHL 1982–2005
DIAG7	How effective is single photon emission computed tomography vs long-term clinical follow-up in determining an accurate diagnosis in patients with a parkinsonian syndrome? * Redone to include differential diagnosis of PD.	Diagnosis	Medline 1966–2005 Embase 1980–2005 Cochrane 1800–2005 CINAHL 1982–2005
DIAG8	How effective is objective smell testing vs long-term clinical follow-up in determining an accurate diagnosis in patients with suspected Parkinson's disease?	All study types	Medline 1966–2005 Embase 1980–2005 Cochrane 1800–2005 CINAHL 1982–2005

continued

Table B1 Details of questions and literature searches – *continued*

Question ID	Question wording	Study type filters used	Database and year
MON1	What is the most appropriate frequency of follow-up after the initial diagnosis of Parkinson's disease?	All study types	Medline 1966–2005 Embase 1980–2005 Cochrane 1800–2005 CINAHL 1982–2005
COMM1	What approach to patient engagement best aids patient understanding on diagnosis of Parkinson's disease?	All study types including qualitative	Medline 1966–2005 Embase 1980–2005 Cochrane 1800–2005 CINAHL 1982–2005 BNI 1985–2005 PsycInfo 1887–2005
TxNP1	Is MAO-B vs placebo or levodopa effective in reducing the rate of progression of early Parkinson's disease?	Systematic reviews, RCTs and comparative studies	Medline 1966–2005 Embase 1980–2005 Cochrane 1800–2005 CINAHL 1982–2005
TxNP2	Are dopamine agonists vs placebo or levodopa effective in reducing the rate of progression of early Parkinson's disease?	Systematic reviews, RCTs and comparative studies	Medline 1966–2005 Embase 1980–2005 Cochrane 1800–2005 CINAHL 1982–2005
TxNP3	Is co-enzyme Q10 vs placebo or levodopa effective in reducing the rate of progression of early Parkinson's disease?	Systematic reviews, RCTs and comparative studies	Medline 1966–2005 Embase 1980–2005 Cochrane 1800–2005 CINAHL 1982–2005 AMED 1985–2005
TxNP4	Are specific vitamins vs placebo or levodopa effective in reducing the rate of progression of early Parkinson's disease?	Systematic reviews, RCTs and comparative studies	Medline 1966–2005 Embase 1980–2005 Cochrane 1800–2005 CINAHL 1982–2005 AMED 1985–2005
TxMN1	What is the effectiveness of MAO-B vs placebo or levodopa in the treatment of early Parkinson's disease?	Systematic reviews, RCTs and comparative studies	Medline 1966–2005 Embase 1980–2005 Cochrane 1800–2005 CINAHL 1982–2005
TxMN2	What is the effectiveness of dopamine-agonists vs placebo or levodopa in the treatment of functionally disabled early Parkinson's disease?	Systematic reviews, RCTs and comparative studies	Medline 1966–2005 Embase 1980–2005 Cochrane 1800–2005 CINAHL 1982–2005
TxMN3	What is the effectiveness of amantadine vs placebo or levodopa in the treatment of functionally disabled early Parkinson's disease?	Systematic reviews, RCTs and comparative studies	Medline 2000–2005 Embase 2000–2005 *Cochrane 2000–2005 CINAHL 2000–2005 *Cochrane search update only

continued

Table B1 Details of questions and literature searches – *continued*

Question ID	Question wording	Study type filters used	Database and year
TxMN4	What is the effectiveness of MAO-B vs dopamine agonists in the treatment of early Parkinson's disease?	Systematic reviews, RCTs and comparative studies	Medline 1966–2005 Embase 1980–2005 Cochrane 1800–2005 CINAHL 1982–2005
TxMN5	What is the effectiveness of immediate-release levodopa vs placebo in the treatment of functionally disabled early Parkinson's disease?	Systematic reviews, RCTs and comparative studies	Medline 1966–2005 Embase 1980–2005 Cochrane 1800–2005 CINAHL 1982–2005
TxMN6	What is the effectiveness of modified-release levodopa vs immediate-release levodopa in the treatment of early Parkinson's disease?	Systematic reviews, RCTs and comparative studies	Medline 1966–2005 Embase 1980–2005 Cochrane 1800–2005 CINAHL 1982–2005
TxMN9	What is the effectiveness of anticholinergics vs placebo in the treatment of functionally disabled early Parkinson's disease?	Systematic reviews, RCTs and comparative studies	Medline 1966–2005 Embase 1980–2005 Cochrane 1800–2005 CINAHL 1982–2005
TxMN10	What is the effectiveness of beta-blockers vs placebo in the treatment of functionally disabled early Parkinson's disease?	Systematic reviews, RCTs and comparative studies	Medline 1966–2005 Embase 1980–2005 Cochrane 1800–2005 CINAHL 1982–2005
TxCM1	What is the effectiveness of adding MAO-B vs placebo in the treatment of later Parkinson's disease patients with motor complications?	Systematic reviews, RCTs and comparative studies	Medline 1966–2005 Embase 1980–2005 Cochrane 1800–2005 CINAHL 1982–2005
TxCM2	What is the effectiveness of adding dopamine-agonists vs placebo in the treatment of later Parkinson's disease patients with motor complications?	Systematic reviews, RCTs and comparative studies	Medline 1966–2005 Embase 1980–2005 Cochrane 1800–2005 CINAHL 1982–2005
TxCM3	What is the effectiveness of adding amantadine vs placebo in the treatment of later Parkinson's disease patients with motor complications?	Systematic reviews, RCTs and comparative studies	Medline 2000–2005 Embase 2000–2005 *Cochrane 2000–2005 CINAHL 2000–2005 *Cochrane search update only
TxCM4	What is the effectiveness of adding dopamine agonists vs MAOB inhibitors in the treatment of later Parkinson's disease patients with motor complications?	Systematic reviews, RCTs and comparative studies	Medline 1966–2005 Embase 1980–2005 Cochrane 1800–2005 CINAHL 1982–2005
TxCM5	What is the effectiveness of adding dopamine-agonists vs amantadine in the treatment of later Parkinson's disease patients with motor complications?	Systematic reviews, RCTs and comparative studies	Medline 1966–2005 Embase 1980–2005 Cochrane 1800–2005 CINAHL 1982–2005

continued

Table B1 Details of questions and literature searches – *continued*

Question ID	Question wording	Study type filters used	Database and year
TxCM6	What is the effectiveness of adding dopamine-agonists vs COMT inhibitors in the treatment of later Parkinson's disease patients with motor complications?	Systematic reviews, RCTs and comparative studies	Medline 1966–2005 Embase 1980–2005 Cochrane 1800–2005 CINAHL 1982–2005
TxCM7	What is the effectiveness of adding COMT inhibitors vs placebo in the treatment of later Parkinson's disease patients with motor complications?	Systematic reviews, RCTs and comparative studies	Medline 1966–2005 Embase 1980–2005 Cochrane 1800–2005 CINAHL 1982–2005
TxCM8	What is the effect of controlled-release levodopa vs immediate-release levodopa in the treatment of later Parkinson's disease?	Systematic reviews, RCTs and comparative studies	Medline 1966–2005 Embase 1980–2005 Cochrane 1800–2005 CINAHL 1982–2005
TxCM9	What is the effectiveness of apomorphine vs standard oral treatment in later Parkinson's disease?	Systematic reviews, RCTs and comparative studies	Medline 1966–2005 Embase 1980–2005 Cochrane 1800–2005 CINAHL 1982–2005
SURG1	What is the effectiveness and safety of any deep brain stimulation procedure vs standard medical therapy in the treatment of motor fluctuations and complications in patients with Parkinson's disease?	All study types	Medline 1966–2005 Embase 1980–2005 Cochrane 1800–2005 CINAHL 1982–2005
SURG2	Which is the most effective form of deep brain stimulation in the treatment of motor fluctuations and complications in patients with Parkinson's disease?	All study types	Medline 1966–2005 Embase 1980–2005 Cochrane 1800–2005 CINAHL 1982–2005
AHP1	What is the effectiveness of physiotherapy vs standard medical therapy or placebo in the treatment of Parkinson's disease?	Systematic reviews, RCTs and comparative studies	Medline 1966–2005 Embase 1980–2005 Cochrane 1800–2005 CINAHL 1982–2005 AMED 1985– 2005
AHP2	What is the effectiveness of speech and language therapy vs standard medical therapy or placebo in the treatment of speech disturbance in Parkinson's disease?	Systematic reviews, RCTs and comparative studies	Medline 1966–2005 Embase 1980–2005 Cochrane 1800–2005 CINAHL 1982–2005 AMED 1985–2005
AHP3	What is the effectiveness of occupational therapy vs standard medical therapy or placebo in the treatment of Parkinson's disease?	Systematic reviews, RCTs and comparative studies	Medline 1966–2005 Embase 1980–2005 Cochrane 1800–2005 CINAHL 1982–2005 AMED 1985–2005

continued

Question ID	Question wording	Study type filters used	Database and year
Table B1 Details of questions and literature searches – *continued*			
AHP4	What is the effectiveness of Parkinson's disease nursing specialist care vs standard care or placebo in the treatment of Parkinson's disease?	Systematic reviews, RCTs and comparative studies	Medline 1966–2005 Embase 1980–2005 Cochrane 1800–2005 CINAHL 1982–2005 AMED 1985–2005 BNI 1985–2005
PSYC1	What is the effectiveness of antidepressant therapies vs placebo or active comparator in the treatment of depression in Parkinson's disease?	Systematic reviews, RCTs and comparative studies	Medline 2001–2005 Embase 2001–2005 *Cochrane 2001–2005 CINAHL 2001–2005 PsycINFO 2001–2005 *Cochrane search update only
PSYC2	What is the effectiveness of atypical antipsychotic therapies vs placebo or active comparator in the treatment of psychosis in patients with Parkinson's disease?	Systematic reviews, RCTs and comparative studies	Medline 1966–2005 Embase 1980–2005 Cochrane 1800–2005 CINAHL 1982–2005 PsycINFO 1887–2005
PSYC3	Is cognitive enhancement therapy effective in dementia in Parkinson's disease and Lewy body dementia?	Systematic reviews, RCTs and comparative studies	Medline 1966–2005 Embase 1980–2005 Cochrane 1800–2005 CINAHL 1982–2005 PsycINFO 1887–2005

Note: The final cut-off date for all searches was 28 February 2005.

Appendix C: Parkinson's Disease Society Communication Table

Table C1 *Communicating with people with Parkinson's and their carers* (2005) (Adapted from Parkinson's Disease Society report[33])	
Principle	**Comment**
General	
Maintain a good knowledge of Parkinson's disease including the symptoms, comorbidities, care and treatment.	All staff who come into contact with people with Parkinson's need to have training and updating on the core symptoms, pharmacology and care.
Use clear language and avoid medical jargon when communicating with people with Parkinson's.	Essential.
Check if the person has understood information provided.	Essential.
Give the person extra time to respond to questions.	Essential.
Ensure information is appropriate, accessible and available in a range of formats.	Essential.
Provide an appropriate setting to communicate, eg a quiet room without interruptions or distractions.	Essential.
Diagnosis	
Communicate the diagnosis in a manner that is sensitive to the needs of the individual, ie if the person wants more information, make this available; if they demonstrate shock or bewilderment, offer a follow-up appointment for further discussion of the symptoms and treatment.	Essential.
Allow extensive opportunities for questions and discussion.	The consultation time should be sufficient to allow for this.
Offer a follow-up discussion.	Essential.
If the consultation reveals a demand for additional specialist information, the person should be referred promptly to the relevant professional (eg Parkinson's nurse, psychiatrist, speech and language therapist, counsellor).	Essential.
Offer written information to supplement the diagnosis. This should include details of specialist organisations such as the Parkinson's Disease Society (PDS).	Essential.
Put the person in contact with specialist support, eg Parkinson's nurse, PDS community support worker. This should include multidisciplinary support (speech and language therapy, physiotherapy, occupational therapy, social workers).	Essential.

continued

Table C1 *Communicating with people with Parkinson's and their carers* (2005). (Adapted from Parkinson's Disease Society report.[33]) – *continued*

Principle	Comment
Diagnosis – continued	
Provide information for carers.	Important but not in all circumstances – the needs of the patient should come first.
Maintenance	
Provide the person with a point of contact for further information.	The PDS recommends that all people with Parkinson's should have access to a PDNS.
Ensure the person has relevant and current information about the condition and treatment specific to their needs and stage of the condition. Provide them with information about all their options, eg medications, home care, therapy.	Essential. Frequency of reviews varies according to the individual but is optimally 6 months. Consultation can take place additionally and in the interim via telephone and email contact.
Consult the person regularly about their physical and emotional needs and financial needs.	Essential.
Consult the carer about the physical and emotional needs of the person they are caring for, and their own support needs.	Essential.
If/when the person goes into hospital, ask them whether they are self medicating, and, if so, facilitate this with access to their drugs at the times prescribed for them.	Essential.
Offer the person access to self-management resources, eg the Expert Patient Programme, if appropriate.	Essential.
Advanced stage care	
Ensure that people and carers receive regular information about the condition, the medications, the financial support and the support networks.	These should be available in a variety of formats, such as print, audio and/or video.
Ensure that staff are aware of the complexities of this stage of the disease and care for their holistic needs and those of their carers including emotional, spiritual and psychological needs.	Essential.

Appendix D: NICE Falls Quick Reference Guide: The assessment and prevention of falls in older people

Key priorities for implementation

▷ Case/risk identification

Older people in contact with healthcare professionals should be asked routinely whether they have fallen in the past year and asked about the frequency, context and characteristics of the fall.

Older people reporting a fall or considered at risk of falling should be observed for balance and gait deficits and considered for their ability to benefit from interventions to improve strength and balance. (Tests of balance and gait commonly used in the UK are detailed in the full guideline.)

▷ Multifactorial falls risk assessment

Older people who present for medical attention because of a fall, or report recurrent falls in the past year, or demonstrate abnormalities of gait and/or balance should be offered a multifactorial falls risk assessment. This assessment should be performed by healthcare professionals with appropriate skills and experience, normally in the setting of a specialist falls service. This assessment should be part of an individualised, multifactorial intervention.

Multifactorial assessment may include the following:
* identification of falls history
* assessment of gait, balance and mobility, and muscle weakness
* assessment of osteoporosis risk
* assessment of the older person's perceived functional ability and fear relating to falling
* assessment of visual impairment
* assessment of cognitive impairment and neurological examination
* assessment of urinary incontinence
* assessment of home hazards
* cardiovascular examination and medication review
* multifactorial interventions.

▷ Multifactorial interventions

All older people with recurrent falls or assessed as being at increased risk of falling should be considered for an individualised multifactorial intervention.

In successful multifactorial intervention programmes the following specific components are common (against a background of the general diagnosis and management of causes and recognised risk factors):

- strength and balance training
- home hazard assessment and intervention
- vision assessment and referral
- medication review with modification/withdrawal.

Following treatment for an injurious fall, older people should be offered a multidisciplinary assessment to identify and address future risk, and individualised intervention aimed at promoting independence and improving physical and psychological function.

▷ Encouraging the participation of older people in falls prevention programmes including education and information giving

Individuals at risk of falling, and their carers, should be offered information orally and in writing about what measures they can take to prevent further falls.

▷ Professional education

All healthcare professionals dealing with patients known to be at risk of falling should develop and maintain basic professional competence in falls assessment and prevention.

Appendix E: Economic modelling – dopamine agonists

Background

Levodopa (LD) remains the mainstay of treatment for PD but with long-term use it causes abnormal involuntary movements (dyskinesias) and fluctuations in motor performance (end-of-dose deterioration and unpredictable 'on/off' fluctuations). To avoid these motor complications, oral dopamine agonists have been used to treat early PD on their own (ie monotherapy).

However, dopamine agonists cost in the region of three times as much as levodopa per year (GDG). The incremental cost-effectiveness of this approach has not been considered in the UK. The large pragmatic PD MED trial will examine the cost effectiveness of these two approaches in the management of early PD.

Aim

The aim of the model was to perform a cost-minimisation analysis based on the assumption of equivalent effectiveness of dopamine agonist versus levodopa therapy in early PD over a 1-year time horizon.

Methods

A cost-minimisation model was constructed from the perspective of the NHS. The effectiveness outcome measure used quality of life. The data sources of the costs and benefits are described in further detail in Tables E1 and E2. No discount rate was used over a 1-year time horizon in accordance with standard practice. A one-way sensitivity analysis was run to assess the impact of variables on the incremental cost of dopamine agonists.

$$\text{Incremental cost} = (C_1 - C_2)$$

Where:

C_1 = Estimated cost of dopamine agonist treatment

C_2 = Estimated cost of levodopa treatment

Data sources and assumptions

Tables E1 and E2 list the baseline cost parameters along with the sources of data. Assumptions and methods of calculating estimates are described in further detail below.

Costs

One study suggests medication costs over a 4-year period are the only cost categories assessed in which there was a statistically significant difference by treatment group (mean = \$8,938 per patient for the pramipexole arm and \$5,399 for the initial levodopa arm, p<0.001).[169] The other cost categories assessed included acute hospitalisations, outpatient provider visits, diagnostic procedures, test and surgeries, emergency department visits, nursing home care, rehabilitation hospital care, durable medical devices, lost wages and home health aid service. Therefore, it was assumed all other cost factors were similar between the alternatives and only the cost of medications were used to compute the incremental costs of dopamine agonist over the levodopa strategy.

Table E1 Mean total daily dosage[158]		
	Levodopa group (N=150)	Dopamine agonist group (N=151)
Experimental dosage	427 ±112 mg (LD)	2.78 ± 1.1 mg/d (salt)
Supplemental LD dosage	274 ± 442 mg	434 ± 498 mg/d

The mean total daily dosage in each alternative was derived from a 4-year RCT comparing pramipexole versus levodopa in initial treatment for PD.[158] In this study, carbidopa/levodopa was taken as 12.5/50 mg or 25/100 mg capsules or matching placebo capsules and pramipexole was taken 3 times per day as 0.25 mg, 0.5 mg or 1 mg salt tablets or matching placebo tablets. Therefore, these tablet sizes were used to derive the unit costs of the medications. The choice of pramipexole as the dopamine agonist was based solely on the clinical reason that it is representative of the class.

The daily cost of the experimental drug therapy and supplemental levodopa was estimated by multiplying the daily dosages in mg with the cost per mg. Total daily cost was the sum of the experimental drug cost and supplemental levodopa cost. Total cost of therapy over one year was calculated as total daily cost multiplied by 365 days.

Additional cost of dopamine agonist treatment

The additional cost of dopamine agonist treatment over a 1-year period was calculated by subtracting the cost of levodopa treatment from the cost of dopamine agonist treatment.

Table E2 Unit costs of medications				
Medication	Cost per mg (£ 2004)	Source	Type	Pack size
Pramipexole	2.467	BNF	180 micrograms base = 250 micrograms salt (0.25 mg)	30-tab pack = £18.50, 100-tab pack = £61.67
	1.963		700 micrograms = 1 mg salt (1 mg)	30-tab pack = £58.89, 100-tab pack = £196.32
Levodopa	0.002	BNF	carbidopa 12.5 mg (as monohydrate), levodopa 50 mg	90-tab pack = £7.03
	0.001		carbidopa 25 mg (as monohydrate), levodopa 100 mg	90-tab pack = £10.05

Effectiveness

The mean change of quality of life scores on both the PDQUALIF and the EuroQoL VAS were not significantly different between the dopamine agonist group and levodopa group and there were no significant treatment differences in the seven subscales of the PDQUALIF in the 4-year randomised control trial.[158] The GDG agreed there was no clear clinically important difference between the two treatment strategies as many dyskinesias are mild and non-disabling and therefore well tolerated by patients. After 4 years of treatment, there is only one additional moderately disabling dyskinesia (1.0%), two mildly disabling dyskinesias (2.0%) and 17 non-disabling dyskinesias (16.8%) in 101 individuals in the levodopa group versus the pramipexole group, whereas the mean improvements in total, motor and activities of daily living UPDRS scores were greater in the levodopa group versus the pramipexole group.[158]

Results

Table E3 Mean total daily cost		
	Levodopa group (£ 2004)	Dopamine agonist group (£ 2004)
Experimental dosage	0.7839 (LD)	6.8573
Supplemental LD dosage	0.3060	0.4846

Table E4 Mean total cost over 1-year period	
Alternative	Cost (£ 2004)
Pramipexole	2,680
Levodopa	286
Incremental cost	2,394

Under the base-case analysis, the additional cost of dopamine agonist treatment versus levodopa over one year is £2,394.

Sensitivity analysis

The estimates used in the model are subject to uncertainty. Therefore, a one-way sensitivity analysis was carried out to assess the impact of key variables using the model. A one-way sensitivity analysis varies one parameter while maintaining the other parameters at base-line values. The variables included are:

(1) unit cost of levodopa
(2) unit cost of pramipexole
(3) mean total daily dosage of experimental levodopa in levodopa treatment
(4) mean total daily dosage of supplemental levodopa in levodopa treatment

(5) mean total daily dosage of experimental pramipexole in pramipexole treatment and

(6) mean total daily dosage of supplemental levodopa in pramipexole treatment.

Results for the upper and lower estimates are given in Table E5. The higher range of the unit cost of levodopa was derived from the higher unit cost of alternative pack size and the lower range was estimated as minus 10%. The lower range of the unit cost of pramipexole was derived from the lower unit cost of alternative pack size and the higher range was estimated as plus 10%. The ranges of the mean total daily dosages were estimated as ± two standard errors derived from the standard deviations and population size in the study.

Table E5 One-way sensitivity analysis

Variable	Baseline value	Range evaluated	Incremental cost with lower range estimate (£ per year)	Incremental cost with higher range estimate (£ per year)
Unit cost of levodopa	0.0011	0.0010–0.0016	2,405	2,351
Unit cost of pramipexole	2.4667	1.963–2.713	1,883	2,644
Mean daily dosage of experimental levodopa	427	409–445	2,402	2,387
Mean daily dosage of supplemental levodopa	274	202–346	2,424	2,365
Mean daily dosage of experimental pramipexole	2.78	2.60–2.96	2,233	2,555
Mean daily dosage of supplemental levodopa	434	353–515	2,361	2,427

The unit cost of pramipexole had the most impact on the ICER and resulted in the widest range of all the incremental cost estimates (£1,883 to £2,644). The mean daily dosage of experimental levodopa had the least impact on incremental cost.

Discussion

The baseline estimates result in an incremental cost (IC) of £2,394 for pramipexole treatment over a 1-year period.

All baseline values were assessed within ranges of uncertainty. The unit cost of pramipexole had the most impact on the IC and resulted in the widest range of all the IC estimates (£1,883 to £2,644). All other variables resulted in a range of incremental costs with an approximate difference of £322 or less between the upper and lower estimates.

This study assumed all other costs, such as acute hospitalisations etc (see 'Costs' under 'Data Sources and assumptions' in this appendix), were similar between the pramipexole and levodopa groups based on the results of an American 4-year study.[169] Evidence of this in the UK setting awaits further research. The study also assumed the quality of life measures are sufficiently sensitive to reflect benefit differences between the alternatives. This study compared initial dopamine agonist therapy with levodopa therapy; however, combination therapy was not included as an alternative.

The model was developed from one RCT based on pramipexole on the basis of available evidence. Other dopamine agonists are currently available and may or may not have similar incremental costs. This is an important consideration as the unit cost of pramipexole had the most impact on the incremental cost.

Conclusion

The baseline estimates result in an incremental cost of £2,394 for pramipexole treatment over a 1-year period. The unit cost of pramipexole had the most impact on the IC and resulted in the widest range of all the IC estimates (£1,883 to £2,644). On the basis of equivalent quality of life between the treatments, the levodopa strategy is the less costly option. The analysis is specific to pramipexole and does not consider the broader range of dopamine agonists available. This model is a simplified version of the costs and benefits of dopamine agonist versus levodopa therapy and a variety of assumptions have been used in the baseline analysis. Therefore, the results should be interpreted with caution.

Appendix F: Economic modelling – surgery

Background

Bilateral subthalamic stimulation has become established for the management of moderate to severe motor complications in the later stages of PD that are unresponsive to changes in medical therapy.

A literature review was performed and four economic studies met quality criteria.[266–269] The economic results are presented along with the clinical evidence of deep brain stimulation.

Whilst conclusive evidence on the cost effectiveness of this procedure awaits the results of ongoing large pragmatic trials in the UK (PD SURG) and US, the GDG considered the topic valuable for further consideration in this guideline.

Aim

The aim of the model was to compare the additional cost of bilateral deep brain stimulation of the subthalamic nucleus (DBS-STN) therapy to the benefits in quality of life gained by this procedure. Treatment option 1 is the intervention: DBS-STN and post-operative care over a 5-year period. Treatment option 2 is standard therapy over a 5-year period. The cost per quality-adjusted life year (QALY) gained was calculated.

Methods

A cost-effectiveness model was constructed from the perspective of the NHS. The effectiveness outcome measure used was quality-adjusted life years (QALYs) and the cost per QALY was calculated. The data sources of the costs and benefits are described in further detail in Tables F1–F4. Costs and benefits were discounted at 3.5% in accordance with current NICE recommendations. A one-way sensitivity analysis was run to assess the impact of variables on the incremental cost-effectiveness ratio (ICER).

$$\text{Incremental cost per QALY} = (C_1 - C_2)/(Q_1 - Q_2)$$

Where:

C_1 = Estimated cost of DBS-STN procedure and post-operative care
C_2 = Estimated cost of standard care
Q_1 = Estimated quality-adjusted life years after DBS-STN
Q_2 = Estimated quality-adjusted life years with no DBS-STN.

Data sources and assumptions

Tables F1–F4 list the baseline cost and effectiveness outcomes along with the sources of data. Assumptions and methods of calculating estimates are described in further detail below.

Table F1 Costs of standard care of PD patients

Cost	Value (£ 1998)	Source
Annual cost of care per patient in Hoehn and Yahr stages III–IV	6,216	Ref 10
Total costs for 5-year period with 3.5% discount	28,066	Estimate

Table F2 Costs of DBS-STN procedure[416]

Item	Minimum (£)	Maximum (£)	Baseline (£)	Quantity
DBS-STN (including device)	12,740	14,450	13,595	1
Follow-up appointment	70	376	223	4
Annual follow-up appointment+	582	582	582	5
Inpatient follow-up for adjustment of stimulator including batteries+	3,000	6,000	4,500	5
Total procedure costs with 3.5% discount+	29,193	45,672	37,432	

+A 3.5% discount rate applies to these figures

Table F3 Costs of post-operative medication

Item	Value	Source
Annual post-operative drug costs per patient	£1,414	Ref 10
% of patients with no medication after DBS-STN	26.19%	Ref 276
Total costs for 5-year period assuming 26.19% with no medication after DBS-STN and 3.5% discount	£4,712	Estimate

Table F4 Benefits after DBS-STN with annual 3.5% discount rate

Year after DBS-STN	Per cent increase in quality of life from initial	Quality of life	Source
Initial	0	0.488	Ref 270
1st year	43	0.673	Ref 270
2nd year	43	0.651	Estimate
3rd year	43	0.629	Estimate
4th year	43	0.607	Estimate
5th year	43	0.587	Estimate
Total potential		3.147	
Total including 7% mortality rate		2.927	

Explanation of assumptions and data used

▷ Costs

Standard care

The annual cost of care per patient with Parkinson's disease in the UK without undergoing DBS-STN was derived from one UK study that estimated the annual cost of care in 1998. The study indicated that Hoehn and Yahr stage significantly influenced cost by stage (p<0.001). Therefore the annual NHS costs in Hoehn and Yahr stages III–IV were averaged to derive the annual standard cost of care of patients with moderate to severe motor complications in the later stages of PD.

To calculate the total cost of care per patient over a 5-year period, the annual cost of care per patient per year is considered stable for the 5-year period and was adjusted by a 3.5% discount rate.

DBS-STN procedure

The cost of the DBS-STN procedure per patient was estimated from cost data obtained from 7 of the 17 centres in the UK offering DBS-STN at the time of the study.[416] Costs of annual follow-up appointment and inpatient follow-up for adjustment of stimulator including batteries after year 1 were discounted at an annual rate of 3.5%. This resulted in a figure similar but conservatively higher (£37,432 (1998) vs £32,526 (2002)) than an estimate in a study assessing the total health service costs of deep brain stimulation of the subthalamic nucleus, including pre-operative assessment, surgery and post-operative management over a 5-year period based on one centre in the UK.[268]

Post-operative medication

The annual post-operative drug costs were derived from the same study used to estimate the cost of standard care.[10] In the study, drug costs were lower in older age groups. The highest drug cost per patient per year in the under 65-year-old age group was used as a conservative estimate in favour of standard care.

The study that estimated the 5-year follow-up of DBS-STN found 11 of the 42 patients no longer required levodopa.[276] Therefore 26.19% (11/42) was used as the baseline value for the percentage of patients no longer requiring medication.

To calculate the cost of post-operative medication per patient over a 5-year period, the annual cost of care per patient per year is considered stable for the 5-year period and was adjusted by a 3.5% discount rate. 26.19% of this cost was subtracted from the result to give the total cost of post-operative medication over the 5-year period.

Total DBS-STN costs

The total cost of the DBS-STN was the sum of the DBS-STN procedure and post-operative medication costs over the 5-year period.

Additional costs of DBS-STN

The additional cost of DBS-STN therapy over a 5-year period was calculated by subtracting the cost of standard care from the cost of DBS-STN therapy.

▷ Quality-adjusted life-years

Standard care

As a conservative estimate in favour of standard care, the study assumed there is no change in quality of life from the initial value over the 5-year period. Quality-adjusted life-years (QALYs) were discounted at 3.5%.

DBS-STN therapy

The initial quality of life and the quality of life 12 months after DBS-STN was derived from one study assessing the quality of life of 60 patients before DBS-STN surgery and 12 months after using a disease-specific quality of life instrument, the PD Quality of Life (PDQL) scale.

There are limited data on the quality of life after DBS-STN beyond the first 12 months and very limited data for converting quality of life outcomes of Parkinson's disease health states, such as UPDRS, into quality-adjusted life-years. Therefore, as UPDRS III has been found to correlate with improvements in QOL,[270] for years 2 through 5, it was assumed that per cent changes in UPDRS III scores correspond with improvements in quality of life. The QoL study found UPDRS III (motor functions) improved by 55% and UPDRS II (activities of daily living) improved by 45% after 12 months. A second study found UPDRS III improved by 54% and UPDRS II improved by 49% after 5 years.[276] Therefore, it was assumed that the quality of life improvements found after 12 months would also remain improved at its 43% increase from baseline after 5 years.

In the UPDRS study[276] over a 5-year follow-up, there was a 7% (3, N=42) rate of mortality, 5% rate of dementia (2, N=42), 19% with eye-lid opening apraxia (8, N=42) and other side effects. To include the 7% mortality, only 93% of the total possible QALY gain was included. The other side effects were assumed to be captured in the quality of life assessment. Total QALY gain in each year was added with a 3.5% annual discount rate.

▷ Results

Table F5 DBS-STN therapy	
Cost	£42,144
QALY	3.147
QALY including 7% mortality	2.927

Table F6 Standard therapy	
Cost	£28,066
QALY	2.203

Table F7 Incremental results of baseline values	
Incremental cost	£14,079
Incremental QALY	0.944
Incremental QALY including 7% mortality	0.723
Incremental cost-effectiveness ratio (ICER)	£14,900 per QALY
ICER including 7% mortality	£19,500 per QALY
Note: Differences due to rounding.	

Under the base-case analysis including 7% mortality, the additional cost is £19,500 per QALY gained.

Sensitivity analysis

The estimates used in the model are subject to uncertainty. Therefore, a one-way sensitivity analysis was carried out to assess the impact of key variables used in the model. A one-way sensitivity analysis varies one parameter while maintaining the other parameters at baseline values. The variables included are:

(1) cost of DBS-STN (including device)

(2) cost of follow-up appointment

(3) cost of inpatient follow-up for adjustment of stimulator including batteries

(4) total costs of DBS-STN procedure with 3.5% discount

(5) drug costs after DBS-STN

(6) total costs of standard care

(7) total QALY gains in standard care

(8) total QALY gains in DBS-STN therapy.

Results for the upper and lower estimates are given in Table F8. The ranges of DBS-STN procedure component costs were derived from the minimum and maximum values given in the cost data literature. The range of the total costs of standard care were estimated from ± two standard errors (867) from the standard deviation (6,235) and sample size of 207 of the annual cost of care. The range of the total DBS-STN procedure cost was estimated as half (× 0.5) and twice (× 2.0) the value. The range of the QALY gains were estimated as ± two standard errors (0.04), from a standard deviation of 0.16 of the per cent increase in quality of life and sample size of 60.

Table F8 One-way sensitivity analysis

Variable	Baseline value	Range evaluated	ICER lower range estimate	ICER higher range estimate	ICER lower range estimate and 7% mortality	ICER upper range estimate and 7% mortality
Cost of DBS-STN (including device)	13,595	12,740–14,450	14,014	15,826	18,282	20,646
Cost of follow-up appointment	223	70–376	14,271	15,568	18,618	20,310
Cost of inpatient follow-up for adjustment of stimulator including batteries	4,500	3,000–6,000	7,743	22,097	10,101	28,826
Total DBS-STN procedure costs with 3.5% discount	37,432	18,716–74,865	6,188	23,652	8,073	30,854
Drug costs after DBS-STN	4,712	3,192–6,384	13,309	16,692	17,362	21,775
% of patients after DBS-STN with no medication	26.19%	50%–0%				
Total costs of standard care	28,066	24,152–31,979	19,067	10,773	24,874	14,054
Annual cost of standard care	6,216	5,349–7,083				
Total QALY gains in standard care	2.203	2.023–2.384	12,523	18,451	15,575	25,940
Total QALY gains in DBS-STN therapy	3.147	2.966–3.328	18,451	12,523		
Total QALY gains in DBS-STN therapy with 7% mortality	2.927	2.759–3.095			25,350	15,796

The total DBS-STN procedure costs with 3.5% discount had the most impact on the ICER and resulted in the widest range of all the ICER estimates (£8,073 to £30,854 per QALY). The cost of DBS-STN (including device) and cost of follow-up appointment had the least impact on the ICER.

Discussion

When possible, the model used conservative estimates that favoured standard care. With these estimates, the ICER value of £19,500 per QALY falls within an accepted range of cost effectiveness. This result is lower than the cost per QALY estimated in the American study –

$49,194 (US$ 2000) per QALY[267] – attributable to methodological and pricing differences between the countries.

Due to the assumptions of UPDRS III and quality of life and the exclusion of side-effects and mortality, the estimate of the QALY gains are associated with the most uncertainty. Nevertheless, the high and low estimates in the sensitivity impact on the ICER resulted in a range of £15,575 to £25,940 per QALY varying QALYs in standard care and £15,796 to £25,350 per QALY varying QALYs after DBS-STN, still falling within a normally accepted range. Even if the improvement in QALY is less than the observed improvement in UPDRS III used to estimate the QALY gain, with the baseline incremental cost of approximately £14,079, only an increase in 0.4693 (achieved by year 3 in baseline analysis) or greater from DBS-STN over a 5-year period would be required to achieve a cost per QALY of £30,000 or less. Doubling the incremental cost of DBS-STN (£28,158) would require an increase in only 0.9386 (achieved by year 5 in baseline analysis) in quality of life or greater to achieve a cost per QALY of £30,000 or less. Therefore, unless the actual total net QALY gain over a 5-year period is less than 0.4693, DBS-STN is still arguably likely to be cost effective.

The benefits in this model are assessed only for a 5-year period. This means that any benefits from DBS-STN accrued after 5 years are not accounted for in the model. This makes each benefit in the 5-year period cost more than it would over time, assuming further benefits after 5 years. Therefore, cost effectiveness may improve over greater lengths of time, but with only small improvements in the ICER. Additionally, the benefits over time are limited by increases in costs of care after DBS-STN as PD progresses and by mortality.

The sensitivity analysis indicates the higher the costs of care of standard therapy, the more favourable the ICER. This may indicate that using DBS-STN in patients with higher costs of care, potentially those with greater severity of PD, is more cost effective, but only if the QALY gains remain the same. Since the higher cost patients may or may not gain on average the same benefits, the sensitivity analysis results do not help to identify those patients better suited to DBS-STN therapy. The lower the cost of the DBS-STN procedure, the more favourable the ICER. This suggests that ICER values will improve if the technology becomes available at lower costs in the future.

Conclusion

Bilateral deep brain stimulation of the subthalamic nucleus is a clinical alternative to standard care for the management of moderate to severe motor complications in the later stages of PD that are unresponsive to changes in medical therapy. Costs and benefits of DBS-STN accrued over greater lengths of time (5 years) in comparison to standard care indicate the potential for cost-effective use of the technology in particular individuals with the clinical potential to benefit from the procedure. The estimate suggests DBS-STN therapy costs approximately £19,500 per QALY over a 5-year period in comparison to standard PD care in the UK (£ 1998). The results are relatively robust based on one-way sensitivity analysis. This model is a simplified version of the costs and benefits of DBS-STN therapy versus standard care and a variety of assumptions have been used in the baseline analysis. Therefore, the results should be interpreted with caution.

Appendix G: Economic modelling for Parkinson's disease nurse specialist care

Background

The Parkinson's Disease Society is encouraging the development of Parkinson's disease nurse specialists (PDNS) across the UK. There are in the region of 180 nurses already in post with plans to increase this to 240 over the next few years (GDG).

A literature search was performed to identify economic evaluations of PDNS care. One study met quality criteria[362] and is presented along with the clinical evidence of Parkinson's disease nurse specialist intervention.

In practice there may be interactions between PDNS care and standard care, which makes it difficult to separate the costs and benefits discretely between the interventions. The GDG considered monitoring medications, as opposed to diagnosing, which is an appropriate example of where PDNS care may substitute standard care with equivalent outcomes. Therefore, the GDG felt it was of value to investigate in this guideline the cost implications of PDNS care based on equivalent effectiveness of completely substituted activities.

Aim

The aim was to estimate the costs and costs saved with equivalently effective and completely substituted PDNS care in comparison to standard care over a 1-year period from the NHS perspective. The additional costs of PDNS care and the cost savings per home visit, per clinic consultation and per hospital-based visit were calculated.

Methods

The annual cost per PDNS was estimated using the sum of the annual salary and training costs discounted at 3.5%. Additional costs of PDNS care were estimated using the unit costs of other professionals' time used in discussing patient care.

Cost savings were estimated from the perspective of the NHS. Estimates were derived from unit costs and discounted at 3.5% (Table G1). Savings were calculated for PDNS care by (a) home visit (b) clinic consultation and (c) hospital-based visit. To calculate savings per intervention, the unit costs of standard care were used to estimate the resources saved by PDNS care.

The net cost of PDNS care over 1 year was calculated as the sum of the annual salary, training costs and additional costs of PDNS care minus the cost savings.

Data sources

Table G1 Unit costs derived from *Unit costs of health and social care 2004*[418]	
Intervention	**Unit cost (£ 2004)**
GP home visit lasting 13.2 minutes (plus 12 minutes travel time)	65
District nurse home visit (A–F)	20
GP clinic consultation lasting 12.6 minutes	28
Nurse practitioner in primary care surgery consultation	14
Hospital-based consultant: per patient-related hour (A–F)	114
Hospital-based staff nurse, 24-hour ward per hour of patient contact	41
Expected annual cost of training at 3.5% discount rate (district nurse)	5,149
Salary per year of district nurse	25,362
Additional cost per visit to GP by PDNS to discuss patient care	28
Additional cost per visit to carer to discuss patient care	0
Additional cost per visit to consultant to discuss patient care	38

A–F: See Ref 418 for definition.

Table G2 Nurse activity – assessing patients[362]	
	Average number or per cent of patients assessed
Per week	13.7
At home	75%
At GP	14%
At hospital consultant clinics	11%

Table G3 Nurse activity – discussing patients[362]	
	Number of visits per week
To GPs	5
To carers	2
To consultants	1

Assumptions

The main assumptions to this costing approach are as follows:

- PDNS care substitutes for standard care for ongoing monitoring of treatment at equivalent effectiveness.
- Nurse activity reflects substituted activities.
- PDNS care is provided at the unit costs and includes the costs for consultant time spent discussing patient care.
- Consultant time is costed per 20-minute visit.

- Healthcare resources for patients by PDNS, such as medication, are similar to standard care.[362]
- Administration activities are included in salary.
- Cost of visit to GP to discuss patient care = cost of nurse time included in salary + cost of GP time = £28.
- Cost of visit to carer to discuss patient care = cost of nurse time included in salary = £0.
- Cost of 20-minute visit to consultant to discuss patient care = cost of nurse time included salary + cost of consultant time = £38.

The results from a randomised control trial suggest PDNS care maintains clinical effectiveness and improves patients' sense of well-being.[362] This supports the assumption that PDNS care has at least equivalent effectiveness to consultant care.

It is not always clear whether PDNS care is substituting some or all of the consultant care or is serving as additional care.[364] In this analysis, consultant care is face-to-face contact with a consultant for PD care needs by a patient. Therefore, the cost-saving estimates pertain only to situations where care is a substitution, such as monitoring medications, and not where the care may be additional to standard care or duplicating standard care.

Results

Table G4 Net cost of PDNS over 1-year period with 3.5% discount rate

Item	Costs (£ 2004)
Cost of training per year	+5,149
Cost of salary per year	+24,504
Additional costs of other health professionals' time discussing patients in one year	+8,974
Cost savings of other health professionals' costs from assessing patients in one year	–39,264
Net cost of PDNS care over one year	–637

Table G5 Additional costs of nurse activity – discussing patient care

	Number of visits per year to discuss patient care[+]	Costs per year (£ 2004)
To GPs	261	7,305
To carers	104	0
To consultants	52	1,983
Total costs		9,288
Total costs at 3.5% discount rate		8,974

[+]Estimated from Table G3 with 1 year = 52.2 weeks.

Table G6 Cost savings of PDNS care when substituting standard care

	Average number of patients assessed[+]	Costs per year (£ 2004)
Per year	714	
At home	536	34,848
At GP	100	2,802
At hospital consultant clinics	79	2,988
Total		40,638
Total costs at 3.5% discount rate		39,264

[+]Estimated from Table G2.

Sensitivity analysis

The estimates used in the model are subject to uncertainty. Therefore, a one-way sensitivity analysis was carried out to assess the impact of key variables used by the model. A one-way sensitivity analysis varies one parameter while maintaining the other parameters at baseline values. The variables included are: (a) cost of training per year, (b) cost of salary per year, (c) additional costs of other health professionals' time discussing patients in one year, and (d) cost savings of other health professionals' costs from assessing patients in one year. Plus or minus 10% was used as an estimate of the variability of the parameters.

Table G7 One-way sensitivity analysis

Variable	Baseline value (£)	Range evaluated	ICER lower range estimate	ICER higher range estimate
Cost of training per year	5,149	4,634–5,664	−1,152	−123
Cost of salary per year	24,504	22,054–26,955	−3,087	+1,813
Additional costs of other health professionals' time discussing patients in one year	8,974	8,076–9,871	−1,535	+260
Cost savings of other health professionals' costs from assessing patients in one year	39,264	35,338–43,190	+3,289	−4,564

− = cost savings
+ = additional cost.

The cost savings of other health professionals' costs had the most impact on the ICER, ranging from an additional cost of £3,289 to cost savings of £4,564. Increasing and decreasing the cost of PDNS training by 10% resulted in cost savings of PDNS. However, by altering the other three parameters, costs range from cost savings to additional costs implying the model is not robust to changes in the assumptions.

Discussion

Based on the average nurse activity in the randomised controlled trial in the UK (Tables G2 and G3),[362] for one year of one PDNS, approximately £640 is saved. Cost savings appear when PDNS care is substituting for standard care. However, in practice there may be variability in the interactions between types of care. There may be substituted care, additional care, duplication of care or a combination of these.[364] Nevertheless, the more PDNS care substitutes for standard care in a practice, the greater the potential for the outcomes to approach these average cost savings. How much PDNS care substitutes, duplicates or increases benefit for the same cost in comparison to standard care is not known. As the sensitivity analysis indicates, the cost savings from other health professionals' costs had the most impact on the ICER ranging from cost savings of £4,564 to an additional cost of £3,289. The costing of other health professionals reflects the average activity of PDNS. Therefore, how much PDNS care is substituting standard care at equivalent effectiveness needs to be assessed in further studies to improve cost estimates.

Only unit costs were used to assess the benefit of PDNS care versus standard care in terms of cost savings. However, unit costs may not fully represent all costs and benefits. This may have under-estimated the benefit of PDNS care. There may be increased patient benefits gained from a greater responsiveness of PDNS care to emerging scientific evidence, such as the earlier reduction in selegiline use found in nurses versus doctors[362] or improved access to care. There may be an improved sense of patient well-being while maintaining clinical effectiveness.[417] There also may be interactions of care as an additional benefit to PDNS care working in standard care that has not been measured. Currently, however, there is insufficient evidence available to measure such benefits.

On the other hand, the unit costs may underestimate the costs of PDNS care. The resources used in PDNS care are assumed to be equivalent to those used in standard care. However, PDNS care may use more or less or higher or lower cost resources resulting in higher or lower costs that are not reflected in the estimate. The RCT is the only study that gives an indication of the cost components in PDNS care versus standard care[362] and suggests that these are similar between the groups. However, apomorphine was excluded from the total cost of healthcare. Therefore, further evidence on the costs of resources used is needed to inform cost-effectiveness analyses.

The initial cost of establishing PDNS care will be incurred by the NHS. Therefore it would be helpful to evaluate whether initial costs can be recovered over time to warrant the initial investment. However, this is also contingent on the resource implications of the care. This cost-savings estimate is based on one PDNS with average nurse activity. While activity with less substitution of standard care or higher resources used would reasonably decrease the cost savings and potentially result in a net cost, it has not been determined how having more than one PDNS would affect costs and cost savings. The net estimate should not be interpreted as the complete indication of the benefit of PDNS care, nor do the estimates provide an indication of the appropriate amount of PDNS care that should be available. Instead, the net estimates suggest on average the cost savings of one PDNS based on average nurse activity.

A sensitivity analysis was performed to investigate changes to the cost inputs used in this analysis on the net cost. Increasing and decreasing the cost of PDNS training by 10% was the only parameter that maintained cost savings of PDNS. Increasing the cost of salary per year and the additional costs of other health professionals' time discussing patients and reducing the cost savings of other health professionals' costs from assessing patients by 10% resulted in additional costs. This suggests that further data are needed to assess the cost effectiveness of PDNS. The baseline analysis pertains to average PDNS care across the UK; however, this does not limit the applicability of the methods to individual centres to assess differences in both costs and cost-savings estimates.

The incremental costs compared with the incremental benefits was not estimated due to the difficulty in separating PDNS care from standard care and the limited evidence on measurable benefits. One study estimated PDNS care costs of £200 per patient per year.[362] However, it is likely this value depends on the total number of patients, PDNSs and nurse activity. Furthermore, PDNS care versus standard care and nurse activity may not be consistent between services. Therefore, cost-effectiveness results may not be generalisable. Due to the difficulty in disentangling PDNS care and consultant care in different practices and the limited measurable benefits, a more general net cost approach, based on completely substituted care with equivalent effectiveness and average nurse activity, was performed.

Conclusion

Increasing the cost of salary per year and the additional costs of other health professionals' time discussing patients and reducing the cost savings of other health professionals' costs from assessing patients by 10% resulted in additional costs. Therefore, the cost effectiveness of PDNS care requires further evidence. This highlights the need for further studies to measure the benefits of PDNS care to adequately assess the cost effectiveness. Due to the interactions of care and data limitations, benefits have been simplified in the form of cost savings from standard unit costs. The cost-saving estimates are subject to the assumptions and therefore the results should be interpreted correspondingly.

Appendix H: Glossary

H.1   Guide to assessment scales

Activities of daily living (ADL)	Measures the impact of PD on 14 categories; each category is scored on a 0–4 scale, with higher scores reflecting greater disability and the need for assistance. The overall score ranges from 0 to 56.
Alzheimer's disease assessment scale – cognitive subscore (ADAS-cog)	A test for measuring cognitive function in people suffering from dementia. The scale can range from 0 to 70, with higher scores indicating more severe impairment and lower scores indicating improvement.
Alzheimer's disease cooperative study – activities of daily living (ADCS-ADL)	A test for measuring quality of life in people suffering from dementia. Scores range from 0 to 78, with higher scores indicating better function.
Alzheimer's disease cooperative study – clinician's global impression of change (ADCS-CGIC)	A test for assessing a change in condition (ie improvement, worsening or no change) of a person suffering from dementia as judged by the clinician. Scores can range from 1 to 7, with a score of 1 indicating marked improvement to a score of 7 indicating marked worsening.
Attitudes to self scale	Measures 'feelings and attitudes towards our bodies/selves'. Consisted of 15 semantic paired opposites (eg tense/relaxed). Positive score was 0 and negative score was 6 (range of total scores 0–90).
Barthel index	Measures the impact of PD on 10 categories of 'activities of daily living'. The range of scores is 0–100 with higher scores indicating better functionality.
Beck depression inventory (BDI)	A test used to measure manifestations and severity of depression. The BDI is a 21-item self-rating scale depression. Each item comprises 4 statements (rated 0–4) describing increasing severity of the abnormality concerned.
Brief psychiatric rating scale (BPRS)	An 18-item scale measuring psychiatric symptoms. Some items can be rated simply on observation; other items involve an element of self-reporting. There are 24 symptom constructs; each rated on a 7-point scale of severity ranging from 'not present' (1) to 'extremely severe' (7).
Clinical global impression (CGI) scale	A participant's illness is compared with change over time, and rated on a scale of very much improved to very much worse. A three-item scale (severity of illness; global improvement; and efficacy index) is used to assess treatment response in participants.

Core assessment program for intracerebral transplantations (CAPIT) dyskinesia rating scale	A pre-operative neurological evaluation. People are evaluated in the 'on' and 'off' phases according to CAPIT protocol. The protocol incorporates UPDRS, a dyskinesia rating scale and timed motor tests to demonstrate efficacy of surgical interventions.
Delis-Kaplan executive function system (D-KEFS) verbal fluency test	Assesses key areas of cognitive function (problem solving, thinking flexibility, fluency, planning, deductive reasoning) in both spatial awareness and verbal communication. Higher scores indicate better performance.
Dementia rating scale (DRS) total score	A test to assess cognitive function in older adults with neurological impairment. The test provides a measurement of attention, initiation, construction, conceptualization, and memory.
Epworth sleepiness scale (ESS)	A subjective scale in which participants rate the likelihood that they will fall asleep or doze in daily sedentary settings (eg watching TV). Each question receives a score of 0 to 3, making the maximum score 24.
EuroQol EQ-5D (VAS)	A questionnaire that provides a simple descriptive profile and a single index value for health status. The questionnaire also includes a visual analogue scale (VAS) to allow the patient to indicate their general health status. On this scale, choosing 100 indicates the best possible health status.
Frenchay dysarthria assessment	A tool developed to diagnose dysarthria by quantitatively evaluating speech across a range of parameters including orofacial muscle movements and a measurement of intelligibility.
Hamilton Rating Scale for Depression (HRSD/HAM-D)	A 17–21 item observer-rated scale to assess the presence and severity of depressive states. A score of 11 is generally regarded as indicative of a diagnosis of depression.
Hoehn and Yahr staging	To establish the severity of PD, stages of disease are classified from I to V where: • I indicates unilateral disease • II indicates bilateral without postural instability • III indicates postural instability • IV indicates considerable disability but ability to walk independently • V indicates wheelchair-bound or walking only with assistance.
Health related quality of life (HRQL)	A combination of a person's physical, mental and social well-being; not merely the absence of disease.

Maintenance of wakefulness test (MWT)	An evaluation of the person's ability to maintain wakefulness for 20-minute periods in a quiet, darkened room with the participant in a reclined position. This test evaluates the person's degree of alertness and his/her tendency to fall asleep at inappropriate times.
Mini-mental state examination (MMSE)	Assessment scale of global cognitive function, with scores ranging from 0 to 30. Higher scores indicate better mental function; <23 is usually indicative of cognitive impairment.
Modified Columbia rating scale (MCRS)	22-item scale (maximum possible score 240) that evaluates parkinsonian and dyskinesia severity, where global disability is rated as 0 (absent) to 4 (severe).
Modified Hoehn and Yahr scale	A modified eight-point version of the original scale.
Montgomery-Asberg depression rating scale	A depression rating scale used to monitor a participant's depressive state over time. Scores range from 0 to 60, with higher scores indicating a greater degree of depression.
Neuropsychiatric inventory 10-item (NPI-10)	A test that evaluates dementia-related behaviours. Scores range from 1 to120, with higher scores indicating more severe or more frequent behavioural problems.
New York University Parkinson's disease scale (NYUPDS)	Determines clinical efficacy by rating participants on 5 symptoms using a 5-point scale ranging from 0 (normal functioning) to 4 (marked impairment).
Northwestern University disability scale (NUDS)	Assessed impairments in activities of daily living on 6 categories, with a scale ranging from 0 (normal functioning) to 10 (marked disability).
Nottingham Health Profile	Generic health-related quality of life measure. The instrument is used to evaluate perceived distress across various populations. There are 38 items with 6 domains. Scores range from 0 to100 where higher scores indicate a greater health problem.
Parkinson's Disease Quality of Life Questionnaire (PDQL)	A questionnaire comprising 37 items addressing four health domains (parkinsonian symptoms, systemic symptoms, social function, and emotional function).
Parkinson's Disease Quality of Life Questionnaire (PDQUALIF)	A questionnaire consisting of 32 questions addressing seven health domains (eg social role, self-image/ sexuality, sleep). The total score ranges from 0 to 128, with lower scores signifying better quality of life.
Parkinson's Disease Questionnaire 39 (PDQ 39)	A self-administered questionnaire, which comprises 39 items addressing eight domains of health, which participants consider to be adversely affected by the disease. Scores range from 0 to 100, where lower scores indicate a better-perceived health status. The results are presented as eight discrete domain scores and not as a total score.

Patient's Global Impression (PGI) scale	A participant rates the change in their illness over time on a scale of '1' very much improved to '7' very much worse.
Positive and Negative Symptoms Scale (PANSS)	A psychotic rating scale of 30 items, each assessed on a seven-point scale from absent to extreme. It is divided into sub-scales covering both positive (PANSS-P) and negative symptoms (N).
Scale for the Assessment of Positive Symptoms (SAPS)	Assesses the severity of psychotic symptoms.
Schwab and England scale ADL (SEADL)	The scale reflects the participant's ability to perform daily activities in terms of speed and independence, and is comprised of 20 points.
Self-assessment Parkinson's Disease Disability Scale (SPDDS)	Participants rate how easy or difficult it was to perform 25 separate actions at their best and at their worst times on a 5-point scale (range of total scores 25 to 125). Higher scores indicate increased difficulty.
Short Form 36 (SF 36)	The SF-36 assesses functioning and well-being in any participant group with chronic disease. Thirty-six items in eight domains are included, which cover functional status, well-being, and overall evaluation of health. Scored range from 0 to 100, where a higher score indicates a better-perceived health status.
Sickness Impact Profile (SIP)	SIP is a general quality of life scale. It consists of 136 items, which measure 12 distinct domains of quality of life. Participants identify those statements, which describe their experience. Higher scores represent greater dysfunction.
Ten-point Clock Drawing Test	A test in which the participant is asked to draw a clock face marking the hours and then draw the hands to indicate a particular time.
Timed-tapping scores	The number of times the participant hits with a finger two spots some 40 cm apart in a 20-second interval.
Trail Making Test	The test consists of two parts. In Part A participants connect, in order, numbers 1–25 in as little time as possible. Part B requires the participant to connect numbers and letters in an alternating pattern (ie 1–A–2–B) in as little time as possible.
Unified Parkinson's Disease Rating Scale (UPDRS)	A scale used to measure severity of Parkinson's disease. It has six parts, and a higher score denotes greater disability.
UPDRS I	Mentation, behaviour, and mood (4 items).
UPDRS II	Activities of daily living (13 items).
UPDRS III	Motor examination (14 items).
UPDRS IV	Complications of treatment (11 items).

UPDRS Total score	Sum total of subscores.
UPDRS V	Modified Hoehn and Yahr staging (8 items).
UPDRS VI	Schwab and England activities of daily living score (20 items).
UPSIT	University of Pennsylvania Smell Identification Test. There are 40 microencapsulated scented pads in a booklet. Each individual scented pad is scratched with a pencil and sniffed one at a time. From a list of 4 choices for each pad, a correct answer must be chosen or a guess made.
Webster Rating Scale	Changes in the scale over time can reflect changes due to disease progression or therapeutic interventions. The scores range from 0 to 30; higher scores indicate greater disease severity.

H.2   Glossary of terms

Adverse events	A harmful, and usually relatively rare, event arising from treatment.
Akinesia	Absence or reduced functionality of movements.
Algorithm (in guidelines)	A flowchart of the clinical decision pathway described in the guideline.
Allied health professional (AHP)	Allied health professionals are involved in the delivery of health services pertaining to the identification, evaluation and prevention of diseases and disorders.
Allocation concealment	The process used to prevent advance knowledge of group assignment in an RCT, and potential bias that may result.
Baseline	The initial set of measurements at the beginning of a study (after run-in period where applicable), with which subsequent results are compared.
Bias	The effect that the results of a study are not an accurate reflection of any trends in the wider population. This may result from flaws in the design of a study or in the analysis of results.
Blinding (masking)	A feature of study design to keep the participants, researchers and outcome assessors unaware of the interventions that have been allocated.
Bradykinesia	Slowness of movement.
Carer (caregiver)	Someone other than a health professional who is involved in caring for a person with a medical condition, such as a relative or spouse.
Clinical audit	A systematic process for setting and monitoring standards of clinical care.

Cochrane Review	A systematic review of the evidence from randomised controlled trials relating to a particular health problem or healthcare intervention, produced by the Cochrane Collaboration.
Cohort	A group of participants.
Confidence interval (CI)	A range of values, which contains the true value for the population with a stated 'confidence' (conventionally 95%).
Control	A person in the comparison group who receives a placebo, no intervention, usual care or another form of care.
Cost-effectiveness analysis (CEA)	An analytic tool in which costs and effects of a programme and at least one alternative are calculated and presented in a ratio of incremental cost to incremental effect. Effects are health outcomes, such as cases of a disease prevented, years of life gained, or quality-adjusted life-years, rather than monetary measures as in cost-benefit analysis.
Cost-minimisation analysis (CMA)	An analytic tool used to compare the net costs of programmes that achieve the same outcome.
Crossover trials	Type of trial comparing two or more interventions in which participants, upon completion of the course of one treatment, are switched to another.
DBS	Deep brain stimulation
Diagnostic study	Any research study aimed at evaluating the utility of a diagnostic procedure.
Differential diagnosis	An attempt to distinguish between two or more diseases with similar symptoms.
Direct costs	The value of all goods, services and other resources that are consumed in the provision of an intervention or in dealing with the side effects or other current and future consequences linked to it.
Discount rate	The interest rate used to compute present value or the interest rate used in discounting future values.
Discounting	The process of converting future values and future health outcomes to their present value.
Disease-modifying therapy	Refers to any treatment that beneficially affects the underlying pathophysiology of PD (also known as 'neuroprotection').
Dysarthria	Slurred or otherwise impaired speech.
Dysarthria profile	A description of the dysarthric person's problems, to supply the speech therapist with indications of where to begin in treatment.

Dyskinesia	The impairment of the power of voluntary movement, resulting in fragmentary or incomplete movements.
Dysphagia	Difficulty in swallowing.
Dystonia	Disordered tonicity of muscle.
Evidence-based healthcare	The process of systematically finding, appraising, and using research findings as the basis for clinical decisions.
Ergot	This is a fungus: *Claviceps purpurea*. Ergot derivatives are nowadays mostly used for their potential to enhance the neurotransmitter, dopamine.
Expert	A qualified medical specialist (see specialist).
False positive	A positive diagnostic test result in a person who does not possess the attribute for which the test is conducted.
FEES	Fibreoptic endoscopic examination of swallow safety.
Follow-up	An attempt to measure the outcomes of an intervention after the intervention has ended.
Generalisability	The degree to which the results of a study or systematic review can be extrapolated to other circumstances, particularly routine healthcare situations in the NHS in England and Wales.
Gold standard	See 'Reference standard'.
Good practice points	Recommended good practice based on the clinical experience of the Guideline Development Group.
Guideline development group (GDG)	An independent group set up by NICE to develop a guideline. They include healthcare professionals and patient/carer representatives.
Hazard ratio (HR)	A statistic to describe the relative risk of complications due to treatment, based on a comparison of event rates.
Heterogeneity	In systematic reviews, heterogeneity refers to variability or differences between studies in estimates of effect.
Homogeneity	In a systematic review, homogeneity means there are no or minor variations in the results between individual studies included in a systematic review.
Hypersomnolence	Excessive sleepiness.
Hypokinesia	Decreased muscular activity, bradykinesia, reduced or slowed movement.
Inclusion criteria	Explicit criteria used to decide which studies should be considered as potential sources of evidence.
Incremental cost	The cost of one alternative less the cost of another.
Incremental cost effectiveness ratio (ICER)	The ratio of the difference in costs between two alternatives to the difference in effectiveness between the same two alternatives.

Intention-to-treat analysis (ITT analysis)	An analysis of the results of a clinical study in which the data are analysed for all study participants as if they had remained in the group to which they were randomised, regardless of whether or not they remained in the study until the end, crossed over to another treatment or received an alternative intervention.
LD	Levodopa.
Lee Silverman Voice Treatment (LSVT)	A treatment for voice and speech disorders associated with Parkinson's disease to improve loudness, voice quality, and articulation.
MAOB inhibitor	Monoamine oxidase type B inhibitor.
Meta-analysis	A statistical technique for combining (pooling) the results of a number of studies that address the same question and report on the same outcomes to produce a summary result.[1]
Mortality	The number of deaths in a given population and during a given time.
Motor fluctuations	Periods of the day with poor or absent motor response to medication alternating with periods of improved motor function.
MSA	Multiple system atrophy.
National Collaborating Centres (NCC)	Professionally led groups established by NICE to harness the expertise of the Royal Medical Colleges, specialist societies and person/carer organisations when developing clinical guidelines.
NCC-CC	National Collaborating Centre for Chronic Conditions.
Negative predictive value	The proportion of people with a negative test result who do not have the disease.
Neuroleptic malignant syndrome	A rare idiosyncratic reaction to neuroleptic medication. The syndrome is characterised by fever, muscular rigidity, altered mental status, and autonomic dysfunction.
NICE	National Institute for Health and Clinical Excellence.
NSF	National service framework.
Odds ratio (OR)	The odds of an event happening in the treatment group, divided by the odds of it happening in the control group.
Off time	The duration of time when anti-parkinsonian medication is not controlling the person's symptoms or is 'wearing-off'.
On time	The duration of time when anti-parkinsonian medication is controlling PD symptoms.

Open label trial design	A clinical trial in which the investigator and participant are aware which intervention is being used for which person. These trials may or may not be randomised.
p values	The probability that an observed difference could have occurred by chance. A p value of less than 0.05 is conventionally considered to be 'statistically significant'.
PD	Parkinson's disease.
PDNS	Parkinson's disease nurse specialist.
PDS	Parkinson's Disease Society.
Phenomenological study	A qualitative study design, the goal of which is to describe a 'lived experience'.
Placebo	An inactive and physically indistinguishable substitute for a medication or procedure, used as a comparator in controlled clinical trials.
Positive predictive value (PPV)	The proportion of people with a positive test result who actually have the disease.
Present value	The value which healthcare professionals and people with PD would attribute at present to an outcome (or avoidance of an outcome) in the future.
PSP	Progressive supranuclear palsy.
Quality of life	Refers to the patient's ability to enjoy normal life activities, sometimes used as an outcome measure in a clinical trial.
Quality-adjusted life-year (QALY)	A measure of health outcome which assigns to each period of time a weighting, ranging from 0 to 1, corresponding to the health-related quality of life during that period, where a weight of 1 corresponds to optimal health, and a weight of 0 corresponds to a health state judged equivalent to death; these are then aggregated across time periods.
Randomisation	Allocation of participants in a study into two or more alternative groups using a chance procedure, such as computer-generated random numbers. This approach is used in an attempt to reduce sources of bias.
Randomised controlled trial (RCT)	A comparative study in which participants are randomly allocated to intervention and control groups and followed up to examine differences in outcomes between the groups.
Reference standard (or gold standard)	The most specific and sensitive test to diagnose a disease or agreed desirable standard treatment and against which other tests or treatments can be compared. An ideal 'gold standard' test would have 100% sensitivity and specificity.

Relative risk (RR)	The number of times more likely or less likely an event is to happen in one group compared with another.
Rigidity	Abnormal stiffness or inflexibility.
Sample size	The number of participants included in a trial or intervention group.
Sensitivity (of a test)	The proportion of people classified as positive by the gold standard who are correctly identified by the study test.
Sensitivity analysis	A measure of the extent to which small changes in parameters and variables affect a result calculated from them. In this guideline, sensitivity analysis is used in health economic modelling.
Sialorrhoea	Increased saliva or drooling.
Single blind study	A study where the investigator is aware of the treatment or intervention the participant is being given, but the participant is unaware.
Somnolence	Sleepiness or unnatural drowsiness.
Specialist	A clinician whose practice is limited to a particular branch of medicine or surgery, especially one who is certified by a higher medical educational organisation.
Specificity (of a test)	The proportion of people classified as negative by the gold standard who are correctly identified by the study test.
Stakeholder	Any national organisation, including patient and carers' groups, healthcare professionals and commercial companies with an interest in the guideline under development.
Statistical power	In clinical trials, the probability of correctly detecting an effect due to the intervention or treatment under consideration. Power is determined by the study design, and in particular, the sample size. Larger sample sizes increase the chance of small effects being detected correctly.
Statistical significance	A result is deemed statistically significant if the probability of the result occurring by chance is less than 1 in 20 ($p<0.05$).
Stereotactic surgery	A precise method of locating deep brain structures by using three-dimensional coordinates. The surgical technique may either involve stimulation or lesioning of the located site.
Systematic review	Research that summarises the evidence on a clearly formulated question according to a pre-defined protocol using systematic and explicit methods to identify, select and appraise relevant studies, and to extract, collate and

report their findings. It may or may not use statistical meta-analysis.

Time horizon	The period of time for which costs and effects are measured in a cost-effectiveness analysis.
Uptake	The absorption of a substance (often a radionucleotide such as Fluoro-dopa) into the brain tissue, which can then be visualised through imaging techniques.
Videofluoroscopy	Videofluoroscopy is a test for assessing the integrity of the oral and pharyngeal stages of the swallowing process. Involves videotaping fluoroscopic images as the patient swallows a bolus of barium.
Washout period	The stage in a crossover trial when one treatment is withdrawn before the second treatment is given.
Withdrawal	When a trial participant discontinues the assigned intervention before completion of the study.

Appendix I: List of registered stakeholders

Addenbrooke's NHS Trust

Age Concern Cymru

Age Concern England

Airedale General Hospital

Alliance Pharmaceuticals Ltd

Amersham Health

Anglesey Local Health Board

Ashfield and Mansfield District PCTs

Association for Continence Advice (ACA)

Association of British Health-Care Industries

Association of British Neurologists

Association of Professional Music Therapists

Association of the British Pharmaceuticals Industry (ABPI)

Barts and the London NHS Trust

Bayer PLC

Birmingham Clinical Trials Unit

Birmingham Heartlands & Solihull NHS Trust

Boehringer Ingelheim Ltd

Bolton, Salford & Trafford Mental Health

Bradford South & West Primary Care Trust

Brain and Spine Foundation

Bristol-Myers Squibb Pharmaceuticals Ltd

Britannia Pharmaceuticals Ltd

British Association for Counselling and Psychotherapy

British Association for Psychopharmacology

British Dietetic Association

British Geriatrics Society

British National Formulary (BNF)

British Neuropsychiatry Association

British Nuclear Medicine Society

British Psychological Society, The

British Society of Neuroradiologists

British Society of Rehabilitation Medicine

BUPA

Cephalon UK Ltd

Chartered Society of Physiotherapy

Cheltenham & Tewkesbury PCT

Cochrane Movement Disorders Group

College of Occupational Therapists

Community District Nurses Association

Community Psychiatric Nurses' Association

Continence Foundation

Co-operative Pharmacy Association

Cyberonics SA/NV

Department of Health

Derbyshire Mental Health Services NHS Trust

Dudley Beacon & Castle Primary Care Trust

Eisai Limited

Elan Pharmaceuticals Ltd

Eli Lilly and Company Ltd

Faculty of Public Health

Gateshead Health NHS Trust

GE Health Care

Gedling Primary Care Trust

GlaxoSmithKline UK

Greater Peterborough Primary Care Partnership-North PCT

Guys & St Thomas NHS Trust

Hammersmith Hospitals NHS Trust

Hampshire Partnership NHS Trust

Healthcare Commission

Help the Aged

Help the Hospices

Hereford Hospital NHS Trust

Herefordshire Primary Care Trust

Hertfordshire Partnership NHS Trust

Independent Healthcare Forum

Institute of Rehabilitation

Institute of Sport and Recreation Management

James Parkinson Centre

Kyowa Hakko UK Ltd

Long Term Medical Conditions Alliance

Lundbeck Limited

Mansfield District PCT

Medeus Pharma Limited

Medicines and Healthcare Products Regulatory Agency (MHRA)

Medtronic Limited

Merck Pharmaceuticals

Mid Staffordshire General Hospitals NHS Trust

National Council for Disabled People, Black, Minority and Ethnic community (Equalities)

National Mental Health Partnership

National Patient Safety Agency

National Public Health Service – Wales

National Schizophrenia Fellowship (Rethink)

National Tremor Foundation

Neurological Alliance

Newcastle, North Tyneside and Northumberland MH Trust

NHS Direct

NHS Health and Social Care Information Centre

NHS Modernisation Agency, The

NHS Quality Improvement Scotland

North Essex Mental Health Partnership Trust

North Staffordshire Combined Healthcare NHS Trust

Novartis Pharmaceuticals UK Ltd

Orion Pharma (UK) Ltd

Orphan Europe UK Ltd

Parkinson's Disease Nurse Specialist Association (PDNSA)

Parkinson's Disease Society

Pfizer Limited

Plymouth Primary Care Trust

Primary Care Neurology Society

Princess Alexandra Hospital NHS Trust

PromoCon (Disabled Living)

Relatives and Residents Association

Roche Products Limited

Royal College of Anaesthetists

Royal College of General Practitioners

Royal College of General Practitioners Wales

Royal College of Nursing (RCN)

Royal College of Physicians of London

Royal College of Psychiatrists

Royal College of Speech and Language Therapists

Royal Pharmaceutical Society of Great Britain

Sanofi-Synthelabo

Schwarz Pharma

Scottish Intercollegiate Guidelines Network (SIGN)

Selby & York PCT

Sheffield Teaching Hospitals NHS Trust

Sherwood Forest Hospitals NHS Trust

Social Care Institute for Excellence (SCIE)

Society of British Neurological Surgeons

Solvay Healthcare Limited

South Birmingham Primary Care Trust

Sue Ryder Care

Teva Pharmaceuticals Ltd

The Medway NHS Trust

The Progressive Supranuclear Palsy [PSP Europe] Association

The Royal Society of Medicine

The Royal West Sussex Trust

Trafford Primary Care Trusts

UK Clinical Pharmacy Association

University College London Hospitals NHS Trust

Valeant Pharmaceuticals

Walton Centre for Neurology and Neurosurgery NHS Trust

Welsh Assembly Government (formerly National Assembly for Wales)

West Cornwall PCT

Wirral Hospital NHS Trust

References

1   National Institute for Health and Clinical Excellence. *Guideline development methods: information for national collaborating centres and guideline developers.* London: National Institute for Health and Clinical Excellence, 2004. Ref ID: 20114

2   Parkinson's Disease Society. *Parkinson's disease: the personal view.* London: Parkinson's Disease Society, 1993. Ref ID: 19909

3   *Dateline* interview: Michael J Fox. New York: NBC News, 2003. Ref ID: 19911

4   Parkinson's Disease Society. *One in twenty: an information pack for younger people with Parkinson's.* London: Parkinson's Disease Society, 2002. Ref ID: 19910

5   Parkinson J. *Essay on the shaking palsy.* London: Sherwood, Neely, and Jones, 1817. Ref ID: 19927

6   Burch B, Sheerin F. Parkinson's disease. *Lancet.* 2005; 365:622-627. Ref ID: 19928

7   Goetz CG. Excerpts from nine case presentations on general neurology delivered at the Salpetriere Hospital in 1887-8. In: Charcot JM (ed), *The Tuesday lessons,* New York: Raven Press, 1987. Ref ID: 19929

8   Dodel RC, Eggert KM, Singer MS et al. Costs of drug treatment in Parkinson's disease. *Movement Disorders.* 1998; 13(2):249-254. Ref ID: 19653

9   Ben-Shlomo Y. The epidemiology of Parkinson's disease. In: Quinn NP (ed), *Parkinsonism.* London: Bailliere-Tindall, 1997: 55-68. Ref ID: 20125

10 Findley L, Aujla M, Bain PG et al. Direct economic impact of Parkinson's disease: A research survey in the United Kingdom. *Movement Disorders.* 2003; 18(10):1139–1145. Ref ID: 40

11 Dodel RC, Berger K, Oertel WH. Health-related quality of life and healthcare utilisation in patients with Parkinson's disease: impact of motor fluctuations and dyskinesias. *Pharmacoeconomics.* 2001; 19(10): 1013–1038. Ref ID: 19691

12 Wood BH, Bilclough JA, Walker RW. Incidence and prediction of falls in Parkinson's disease: a prospective multidisciplinary study. *Journal of Neurology, Neurosurgery & Psychiatry.* 2002; 72:721–725. Ref ID: 19857

13 National Institute for Health and Clinical Excellence. *Guideline development methods: an overview for stakeholders, the public and the NHS.* London: National Institute for Health and Clinical Excellence, 2004. Ref ID: 20115

14 Department of Health. *The national service framework for long-term (neurological) conditions.* London: HMSO, 2005. Ref ID: 19904

15 Department of Health. *The national service framework for older people.* London: HMSO, 2001. Ref ID: 19942

16 National Institute for Health and Clinical Excellence. *Falls: The assessment and prevention of falls in older people.* (Clinical Guideline 21). London: National Institute for Health and Clinical Excellence, 2004. Ref ID: 19925

17 National Institute for Health and Clinical Excellence and Social Care Institute for Excellence. *Dementia: management of dementia, including use of antipsychotic medication in older people (In progress).* London: National Institute for Health and Clinical Excellence, 2007. Ref ID: 19926

18 National Institute for Clinical Excellence. *Depression: management of depression in primary and secondary care.* (Clinical Guideline 23). London: National Institute for Clinical Excellence, 2004. Ref ID: 19852

19 National Institute for Clinical Excellence. *The epilepsies: the diagnosis and management of the epilepsies in adults and children in primary and secondary care.* (Clinical Guideline 20). London: National Institute for Clinical Excellence, 2004. Ref ID: 20031

20 National Institute for Clinical Excellence. *Guidance on the use of donepezil, rivastigmine and galantamine for the treatment of Alzheimer's disease.* (Technology Appraisal Guidance 19). London: National Institute for Clinical Excellence, 2001. Ref ID: 19943

21   National Institute for Clinical Excellence. *Anxiety: management of anxiety (panic disorder, with or without agoraphobia, and generalised anxiety disorder) in adults in primary, secondary and community care.* (Clinical Guideline 22). London: National Institute for Clinical Excellence, 2004. Ref ID: 19941

22   National Institute for Clinical and Public Health Excellence. *Nutrition support in adults: oral nutrition support, enteral tube feeding and parenteral nutrition.* (Clinical Guideline 32). London: National Institute for Clinical and Public Health Excellence, 2006. Ref ID: 20124

23   National Institute for Clinical Excellence. *Deep brain stimulation for Parkinson's disease.* (IPG019). London: NICE, 2003. Ref ID: 95

24   National Collaborating Centre for Chronic Conditions. *Methodology pack.* London: NCC-CC, 2006. Available from: www.rcplondon.ac.uk/college/NCC-CC. Ref ID: 20117

25   Department of Health. *The expert patient: a new approach to chronic disease management for the 21st century.* London: Department of Health, 2001. Ref ID: 19595

26   Montgomery EB, Lieberman A, Singh G et al. Patient education and health promotion can be effective in Parkinson's disease: a randomized controlled trial. PROPATH Advisory Board. *American Journal of Medicine.* 1994; 97(5):429–435. Ref ID: 737

27   Mercer BS. A randomized study of the efficacy of the PROPATH program for patients with Parkinson disease. *Archives of Neurology.* 1996; 53:881–884. Ref ID: 739

28   Findley L, Eichhorn T, Janca A et al. Factors impacting on quality of life in Parkinson's disease: results from an international survey. *Movement Disorders.* 2002; 17(1):60–67. Ref ID: 742

29   Habermann B. Day-to-day demands of Parkinson's disease. *Western Journal of Nursing Research.* 1996; 18(4):397–413. Ref ID: 65

30   Pentland B, Pitkairn TK, Gray TK. The effects of reduced expression in Parkinson's disease in impression formation by health professionals. *Clinical Rehabilitation.* 1987; 1:307–313. Ref ID: 2766

31   Yarrow, S. *Survey of members of the Parkinson's Disease Society.* London: Parkinson's Disease Society of the United Kingdom and Policy Studies Institute, 1999. Ref ID: 786

32   Shimbo T, Goto M, Morimoto T et al. Association between patient education and health-related quality of life in patients with Parkinson's disease. *Quality of Life Research.* 2004; 13(1):81–89. Ref ID: 19841

33   Meadowcroft RS, Scott S, and Woodford C. *Communicating with people with Parkinson's and their carers.* London: Parkinson's Disease Society, 2005. Ref ID: 19903

34   Bennett DA, Beckett AM, Shannon KM et al. Prevalence of parkinsonian signs and associated mortality in a community population of older people. *New England Journal of Medicine.* 1996; 334(24):71–76. Ref ID: 2772

35   Gibb WRG, Lees AJ. The relevance of the Lewy body to the pathogenesis of idiopathic Parkinson's disease. *Journal of Neurology, Neurosurgery & Psychiatry.* 1988; 51(6):745–752. Ref ID: 2773

36   Rajput AH, Rozdilsky B, Rajput A. Accuracy of clinical diagnosis in Parkinsonism - A prospective study. *Canadian Journal of Neurological Sciences.* 1991; 18(3):275–278. Ref ID: 111

37   Hughes AJ, Daniel SE, Kilford L et al. Accuracy of clinical diagnosis of idiopathic Parkinson's disease: a clinico-pathological study of 100 cases. *Journal of Neurology, Neurosurgery & Psychiatry.* 1992; 55(3): 181–184. Ref ID: 99

38   Hughes AJ, Daniel SE, Ben Shlomo Y et al. The accuracy of diagnosis of parkinsonian syndromes in a specialist movement disorder service. *Brain.* 2002; 125(Pt:4):4–70. Ref ID: 96

39   Schrag A, Ben Shlomo Y, Quinn N. How valid is the clinical diagnosis of Parkinson's disease in the community? *Journal of Neurology, Neurosurgery & Psychiatry.* 2002; 73(5):529–534. Ref ID: 142

40   Meara J, Bhowmick BK, Hobson P. Accuracy of diagnosis in patients with presumed Parkinson's disease. *Age & Ageing.* 1999; 28(2):99–102. Ref ID: 108

41   Jankovic J, Rajput AH, McDermott MP et al. The evolution of diagnosis in early Parkinson disease. *Archives of Neurology.* 2000; 57(3):369–372. Ref ID: 81

42   Lees AJ, Katzenschlager R, Head J et al. Ten-year follow-up of three different initial treatments in de-novo PD: a randomized trial. *Neurology.* 2001; 57(9):1687–1694. Ref ID: 2309

43 Benamer HT, Oertel WH, Patterson J et al. Prospective study of presynaptic dopaminergic imaging in patients with mild parkinsonism and tremor disorders: part 1. Baseline and 3-month observations. *Movement Disorders.* 2003; 18(9):977–984. Ref ID: 425

44 Popperl G, Radau P, Linke R et al. Diagnostic performance of a 3-D automated quantification method of dopamine D2 receptor SPECT studies in the differential diagnosis of parkinsonism. *Nuclear Medicine Communications.* 2005; 26(1):39–43. Ref ID: 19822

45 Benamer TS, Patterson J, Grosset DG et al. Accurate differentiation of parkinsonism and essential tremor using visual assessment of [123I]-FP-CIT SPECT imaging: the [123I]-FP-CIT study group. *Movement Disorders.* 2000; 15(3):503–510. Ref ID: 484

46 Booij J, Speelman JD, Horstink MW et al. The clinical benefit of imaging striatal dopamine transporters with [123I]FP-CIT SPET in differentiating patients with presynaptic parkinsonism from those with other forms of parkinsonism. *European Journal of Nuclear Medicine.* 2001; 28(3):266–272. Ref ID: 467

47 Lokkegaard A, Werdelin LM, Friberg L. Clinical impact of diagnostic SPET investigations with a dopamine re-uptake ligand. *European Journal of Nuclear Medicine & Molecular Imaging.* 2002; 29(12):1623–1629. Ref ID: 439

48 Prunier C, Tranquart F, Cottier JP et al. Quantitative analysis of striatal dopamine D2 receptors with 123 I-iodolisuride SPECT in degenerative extrapyramidal diseases. *Nuclear Medicine Communications.* 2001; 22(11):1207–1214. Ref ID: 459

49 Parkinson Study Group. A multicenter assessment of dopamine transporter imaging with DOPASCAN/SPECT in parkinsonism. *Neurology.* 2000; 55(10):1540–1547. Ref ID: 475

50 Van Laere K, De Ceuninck L, Dom R et al. Dopamine transporter SPECT using fast kinetic ligands: 123I-FP- beta-CIT versus 99mTc-TRODAT-1. *European Journal of Nuclear Medicine & Molecular Imaging.* 2004; 31(8):1119–1127. Ref ID: 19824

51 Chou KL, Hurtig HI, Stern MB et al. Diagnostic accuracy of [99mTc]TRODAT-1 SPECT imaging in early Parkinson's disease. *Parkinsonism & Related Disorders.* 2004; 10(6):375–379. Ref ID: 19817

52 Asenbaum S, Pirker W, Angelberger P et al. [123I]beta-CIT and SPECT in essential tremor and Parkinson's disease. *Journal of Neural Transmission.* 1998; 105(10-12):1213–1228. Ref ID: 507

53 Acton PD, Mozley PD, Kung HF. Logistic discriminant parametric mapping: a novel method for the pixel-based differential diagnosis of Parkinson's disease. *European Journal of Nuclear Medicine.* 1999; 26(11): 1413–1423. Ref ID: 196

54 Varrone A, Marek KL, Jennings D et al. [123I]beta-CIT SPECT imaging demonstrates reduced density of striatal dopamine transporters in Parkinson's disease and multiple system atrophy. *Movement Disorders.* 2001; 16(6):1023–1032. Ref ID: 453

55 Huang WS, Lee MS, Lin JC et al. Usefulness of brain 99mTc-TRODAT-1 SPET for the evaluation of Parkinson's disease. *European Journal of Nuclear Medicine & Molecular Imaging.* 2004; 31(2):155–161. Ref ID: 19820

56 Catafau AM, Tolosa E, Laloux P et al. Impact of dopamine transporter SPECT using 123I-Ioflupane on diagnosis and management of patients with clinically uncertain parkinsonian syndromes. *Movement Disorders.* 2004; 19(10):1175–1182. Ref ID: 19823

57 Weng YH, Yen TC, Chen MC et al. Sensitivity and specificity of 99mTc-TRODAT-1 SPECT imaging in differentiating patients with idiopathic Parkinson's disease from healthy subjects. *Journal of Nuclear Medicine.* 2004; 45(3):393–401. Ref ID: 19821

58 Jennings DL, Seibyl JP, Oakes D et al. [123I]beta-CIT and single-photon emission computed tomographic imaging vs clinical evaluation in Parkinsonian syndrome: unmasking an early diagnosis. *Archives of Neurology.* 2004; 61(8):1224–1229. Ref ID: 19818

59 Dodel RC, Hoffken H, Moller JC et al. Dopamine transporter imaging and SPECT in diagnostic work-up of Parkinson's disease: a decision-analytic approach. *Movement Disorders.* 2003; 18(Suppl 7):S52–S62. Ref ID: 19666

60 Holloway R, Shoulson I, Kieburtz K et al. Pramipexole vs levodopa as initial treatment for Parkinson disease: a randomized controlled trial. *Journal of the American Medical Association.* 2000; 284(15): 1931–1938. Ref ID: 1477

61 Whone AL, Watts RL, Stoessl AJ et al. Slower progression of Parkinson's disease with ropinirole versus levodopa: The REAL-PET study. *Annals of Neurology.* 2003; 54(1):93–101. Ref ID: 808

62 Fahn S, Oakes D, Shoulson I et al. Levodopa and the progression of Parkinson's disease. *New England Journal of Medicine.* 2004; 351(24):2498–2508. Ref ID: 19725

63 Burn DJ, Sawle GV, Brooks DJ. Differential diagnosis of Parkinson's disease, multiple system atrophy, and Steele-Richardson-Olszewski syndrome: discriminant analysis of striatal 18F-dopa PET data. *Journal of Neurology, Neurosurgery & Psychiatry.* 1994; 57(3):278–284. Ref ID: 329

64 Schocke MFH, Seppi K, Esterhammer R et al. Diffusion-weighted MRI differentiates the Parkinson variant of multiple system atrophy from PD. *Neurology.* 2002; 58(4):575–580. Ref ID: 130

65 Cercy SP, Bylsma FW. Lewy bodies and progressive dementia: A critical review and meta-analysis. *Journal of the International Neuropsychological Society.* 1997; 3(2):179–194. Ref ID: 29

66 Bhattacharya K, Saadia D, Eisenkraft B et al. Brain magnetic resonance imaging in multiple-system atrophy and Parkinson disease: A diagnostic algorithm. *Archives of Neurology.* 2002; 59(5):835-842. Ref ID: 13

67 Juh R, Kim J, Moon D et al. Different metabolic patterns analysis of Parkinsonism on the 18F-FDG PET. *European Journal of Radiology.* 2004; 51(3):223-233. Ref ID: 19839

68 Schreckenberger M, Hagele S, Siessmeier T et al. The dopamine D2 receptor ligand 18F-desmethoxy-fallypride: An appropriate fluorinated PET tracer for the differential diagnosis of parkinsonism. *European Journal of Nuclear Medicine & Molecular Imaging.* 2004; 31(8):1128–1135. Ref ID: 19838

69 Eidelberg D, Moeller JR, Ishikawa T et al. Early differential diagnosis of Parkinson's disease with 18F-fluorodeoxyglucose and positron emission tomography. *Neurology.* 1995; 45(11):1995–2004. Ref ID: 291

70 Sawle GV, Playford ED, Burn DJ et al. Separating Parkinson's disease from normality. Discriminant function analysis of fluorodopa F 18 positron emission tomography data. *Archives of Neurology.* 1994; 51(3):237–243. Ref ID: 213

71 Righini A, Antonini A, Ferrarini M et al. Thin section MR study of the basal ganglia in the differential diagnosis between striatonigral degeneration and Parkinson disease. *Journal of Computer Assisted Tomography.* 2002; 26(2):266–271. Ref ID: 129

72 Seppi K, Schocke MFH, Esterhammer R et al. Diffusion-weighted imaging discriminates progressive supranuclear palsy from PD, but not from the parkinson variant of multiple system atrophy. *Neurology.* 2003; 60(6):922–927. Ref ID: 133

73 Yekhlef F, Ballan G, Macia F et al. Routine MRI for the differential diagnosis of Parkinson's disease, MSA, PSP, and CBD. *Journal of Neural Transmission.* 2003; 110(2):151–169. Ref ID: 135

74 Price S, Paviour D, Scahill R et al. Voxel-based morphometry detects patterns of atrophy that help differentiate progressive supranuclear palsy and Parkinson's disease. *Neuroimage.* 2004; 23(2):663–669. Ref ID: 19826

75 Righini A, Antonini A, De Notaris R et al. MR imaging of the superior profile of the midbrain: Differential diagnosis between progressive supranuclear palsy and Parkinson disease. *American Journal of Neuroradiology.* 2004; 25(6):927–932. Ref ID: 19827

76 Paviour DC, Price SL, Stevens JM et al. Quantitative MRI measurement of superior cerebellar peduncle in progressive supranuclear palsy. *Neurology.* 2005; 64(4):675–679. Ref ID: 19831

77 Cordato NJ, Pantelis C, Halliday GM et al. Frontal atrophy correlates with behavioural changes in progressive supranuclear palsy. *Brain.* 2002; 125(4):789–800. Ref ID: 123

78 Clarke CE, Lowry M. Systematic review of proton magnetic resonance spectroscopy of the striatum in parkinsonian syndromes. *European Journal of Neurology.* 2001; 8(6):573–577. Ref ID: 17

79 Clarke CE, Davies P. Systematic review of acute levodopa and apomorphine challenge tests in the diagnosis of idiopathic Parkinson's disease. *Journal of Neurology, Neurosurgery & Psychiatry.* 2000; 69(5):590–594. Ref ID: 21

80   Rossi P, Colosimo C, Moro E et al. Acute challenge with apomorphine and levodopa in Parkinsonism. *European Neurology.* 2000; 43(2):95–101. Ref ID: 719

81   Hughes AJ. Apomorphine test in the assessment of parkinsonian patients: a meta-analysis. *Advances in Neurology.* 1999; 80:363–368. Ref ID: 720

82   Hughes AJ, Lees AJ, Stern GM. Apomorphine test to predict dopaminergic responsiveness in parkinsonian syndromes. *Lancet.* 1990; 336(8706):32–34. Ref ID: 84

83   D'Costa DF, Abbott RJ, Pye IF et al. The apomorphine test in parkinsonian syndromes. *Journal of Neurology, Neurosurgery & Psychiatry.* 1991; 54(10):870–872. Ref ID: 79

84   Zappia M, Montesanti R, Colao R et al. Short-term levodopa test assessed by movement time accurately predicts dopaminergic responsiveness in Parkinson's disease. *Movement Disorders.* 1997; 12(1):103–106. Ref ID: 731

85   Double KL, Rowe DB, Hayes M et al. Identifying the pattern of olfactory deficits in Parkinson disease using the brief smell identification test. *Archives of Neurology.* 2003; 60(4):545–549. Ref ID: 699

86   Muller A, Mungersdorf M, Reichmann H et al. Olfactory function in Parkinsonian syndromes. *Journal of Clinical Neuroscience.* 2002; 9(5):521–524. Ref ID: 700

87   Wenning GK, Shephard B, Hawkes C et al. Olfactory function in atypical parkinsonian syndromes. *Acta Neurologica Scandinavica.* 1995; 91(4):247–250. Ref ID: 707

88   Antonini A, Benti R, De Notaris R et al. 123I-ioflupane/SPECT binding to striatal dopamine transporter (DAT) uptake in patients with Parkinson's disease, multiple system atrophy, and progressive supranuclear palsy. *Neurological Sciences.* 2003; 24(3):149–150. Ref ID: 789

89   Hawkes CH, Shephard BC, Daniel SE. Olfactory dysfunction in Parkinson's disease. *Journal of Neurology, Neurosurgery & Psychiatry.* 1997; 62(5):436–446. Ref ID: 703

90   Doty RL, Bromley SM, Stern MB. Olfactory testing as an aid in the diagnosis of Parkinson's disease: development of optimal discrimination criteria. *Neurodegeneration.* 1995; 4(1):93–97. Ref ID: 708

91   Katzenschlager R, Zijlmans J, Evans A et al. Olfactory function distinguishes vascular parkinsonism from Parkinson's disease. *Journal of Neurology, Neurosurgery & Psychiatry.* 2004; 75(12):1749–1752. Ref ID: 19807

92   Mesholam RI, Moberg PJ, Mahr RN et al. Olfaction in neurodegenerative disease: a meta-analysis of olfactory functioning in Alzheimer's and Parkinson's diseases. *Archives of Neurology.* 1998; 55(1):84–90. Ref ID: 702

93   Mitchell A, Lewis S, Foltynie T et al. Biomarkers and Parkinson's disease. *Brain.* 2004; 127:1693–1705. Ref ID: 19536

94   Clarke CE. A 'cure' for Parkinson's disease: can neuroprotection be proven with current trial designs? *Movement Disorders.* 2004; 19:491–499. Ref ID: 19538

95   Clarke CE. *Parkinson's disease in practice.* London: Royal Society of Medicine Press, 2001. Ref ID: 2

96   Schapira A. Disease modification in Parkinson's disease. *Lancet Neurology.* 2004; 3:362–368. Ref ID: 19537

97   Clarke CE, Guttman M. Dopamine agonist monotherapy in Parkinson's disease. *Lancet.* 2002; 360(9347):1767–1769. Ref ID: 16

98   Clarke CE. Neuroprotection and pharmacotherapy for motor symptoms in Parkinson's disease. *Lancet Neurology.* 2004; 3:466–475. Ref ID: 19540

99   Parkinson Study Group. A controlled, randomized, delayed-start study of rasagiline in early Parkinson disease. *Archives of Neurology.* 2004; 61(4):561–566. Ref ID: 2764

100   Ravina BM, Fagan SC, Hart RG. Neuroprotective agents for clinical trials in Parkinson's disease. *Neurology.* 2003; 60:1234–1240. Ref ID: 19541

101   Shults CW. Effect of selegiline (deprenyl) on the progression of disability in early Parkinson's disease. Parkinson Study Group. *Acta Neurologica Scandinavica Supplementum.* 1993; 146:36–42. Ref ID: 805

102   Kieburtz K, McDermott M, Como P et al. The effect of deprenyl and tocopherol on cognitive performance in early untreated Parkinson's disease. *Neurology.* 1994; 44(9):1756–1759. Ref ID: 281

103   Koller W, Olanow CW, Rodnitzky R et al. Effects of tocopherol and deprenyl on the progression of disability in early Parkinson's disease. *New England Journal of Medicine.* 1993; 328(3):176–183. Ref ID: 148

104   Shoulson I. Deprenyl and tocopherol antioxidative therapy of parkinsonism (DATATOP). *Acta Neurologica Scandinavica Supplementum.* 1989; 80(126):171–175. Ref ID: 363

105   Parker W, Boyson S, Parks J. Abnormalities of the electron transport chain in idiopathic Parkinson's disease. *Annals of Neurology.* 1989; 26:719–723. Ref ID: 19543

106   Schapira A, Mann V, Cooper J. Anatomic and disease specificity of NADH CoQ1 reductase (complex 1) deficiency in Parkinson's disease. *Journal of Neurochemistry.* 1990; 55:2142–2145. Ref ID: 19544

107   Shults C, Haas R, Passov D et al. Coenzyme Q10 levels correlate with the activities of the complex I and II/III mitochrondria from parkinsonian and non-parkinsonian subjects. *Annals of Neurology.* 1997; 42:261–264. Ref ID: 19545

108   Beal MF, Matthews R, Tieleman A et al. Coenzyme Q10 attenuates the MPTP induced loss of striatal dopamine and dopaminergic axons in aged mice. *Brain Research.* 1998; 783:109–114. Ref ID: 19546

109   Muller T, Buttner T, Gholipour AF et al. Coenzyme Q10 supplementation provides mild symptomatic benefit in patients with Parkinson's disease. *Neuroscience Letters.* 2003; 341(3):201–204. Ref ID: 799

110   Shults CW, Oakes D, Kieburtz K et al. Effects of coenzyme Q10 in early Parkinson disease: evidence of slowing of the functional decline. *Archives of Neurology.* 2002; 59(10):1541–1550. Ref ID: 801

111   Lida M, Miyazaki I, Tanaka K et al. Dopamine D2 receptor-mediated antioxidant and neuroprotective effects of ropinirole, a dopamine agonist. *Brain Research.* 1999; 838:51–59. Ref ID: 19547

112   Schapira A, Olanow CW. Rationale for the use of dopamine agonists as neuroprotective agents in Parkinson's disease. *Annals of Neurology.* 2003; 53:S149–S157. Ref ID: 19549

113   Marek K. Dopamine transporter brain imaging to assess the effects of pramipexole vs levodopa on Parkinson disease progression. *Journal of the American Medical Association.* 2002; 287(13):1653–1661. Ref ID: 809

114   Rakshi JS, Pavese N, Uema T et al. A comparison of the progression of early Parkinson's disease in patients started on ropinirole or L-dopa: an 18F-dopa PET study. *Journal of Neural Transmission.* 2002; 109(12):1433–1443. Ref ID: 2535

115   Przuntek H, Welzel D, Blumner E et al. Bromocriptine lessens the incidence of mortality in L-dopa-treated parkinsonian patients: prado-study discontinued. *European Journal of Clinical Pharmacology.* 1992; 43(4):357–363. Ref ID: 2518

116   Hely MA, Morris JG, Traficante R et al. The sydney multicentre study of Parkinson's disease: progression and mortality at 10 years. *Journal of Neurology, Neurosurgery & Psychiatry.* 1999; 67(3):300–307. Ref ID: 2184

117   Montastruc JL, Desboeuf K, Lapeyre-Mestre M et al. Long-term mortality results of the randomized controlled study comparing bromocriptine to which levodopa was later added with levodopa alone in previously untreated patients with Parkinson's disease. *Movement Disorders.* 2001; 16(3):511–514. Ref ID: 2414

118   Rinne UK, Bracco F, Chouza C et al. Early treatment of Parkinson's disease with Cabergoline delays the onset of motor complications. Results of a double-blind levodopa controlled trial. *Drugs.* 1998; 55(Suppl 1):23–3TxCM 20. Ref ID: 19605

119   Hundemer HP, Lledo A, Van Laar T et al. The safety of pergolide monotherapy in early stage Parkinson's disease. One year interim analysis of a 3 year double blind randomised study of pergolide versus levodopa (abstract). *Movement Disorders.* 2000; 15(Supplement 3):115. Ref ID: 19598

120   Ives NJ, Stowe RL, Marro J et al. Monoamine oxidase type B inhibitors in early Parkinsons's disease: meta analysis of 17 randomised trials involving 3525 patients. *British Medical Journal.* 2004; 329(7466):593–596. Ref ID: 2739

121   Macleod AD, Counsell CE, Ives N et al. Monoamine oxidase B inhibitors for early Parkinson's disease. *The Cochrane Database of Systematic Reviews.* 2005;(3):CD004898. Ref ID: 20026

122 Barone P, Bravi D, Bermejo-Pareja F et al. Pergolide monotherapy in the treatment of early PD: a randomized, controlled study. Pergolide Monotherapy Study Group. *Neurology.* 1999; 53(3):573–579. Ref ID: 1937

123 Kieburtz K. Safety and efficacy of pramipexole in early Parkinson disease: A randomized dose-ranging study. *Journal of the American Medical Association.* 1997; 278(2):125–130. Ref ID: 1501

124 Adler CH, Sethi KD, Hauser RA et al. Ropinirole for the treatment of early Parkinson's disease. *Neurology.* 1997; 49(2):393–399. Ref ID: 1902

125 Shannon KM, Bennett JPJ, Friedman JH. Efficacy of pramipexole, a novel dopamine agonist, as monotherapy in mild to moderate Parkinson's disease. *Neurology.* 1997; 49(3):724–728. Ref ID: 19764

126 Hubble JP, Koller WC, Cutler NR et al. Pramipexole in patients with early Parkinson's disease. *Clinical Neuropharmacology.* 1995; 18(4):338–347. Ref ID: 19643

127 Brooks DJ, Abbott RJ, Lees AJ et al. A placebo-controlled evaluation of ropinirole, a novel D2 agonist, as sole dopaminergic therapy in Parkinson's disease. *Clinical Neuropharmacology.* 1998; 21(2):101–107. Ref ID: 1977

128 Committee on Safety of Medicines. Fibrotic reactions with pergolide and other ergot-derived dopamine receptor agonists. *Current Problems in Pharmacovigilance.* 2002; 28(3) Ref ID: 19899

129 Baseman D, O'Suilleabhain P. Pergolide use in Parkinson's disease is associated with cardiac valve regurgitation. *Neurology.* 2004; 63:301–304. Ref ID: 19900

130 Van Camp G, Flamez A. Treatment of Parkinson's disease with pergolide and relation to restrictive valvular heart disease. *Lancet.* 2004; 363:1179–1183. Ref ID: 19901

131 Birkmayer W, Knoll J, Riederer P et al. Increased life expectancy resulting from addition of L-deprenyl to madopar treatment in Parkinson's disease: a long-term study. *Journal of Neural Transmission.* 1985; 64:113–127. Ref ID: 19677

132 Stern MB, Marek KL, Friedman J et al. Double-blind, randomized, controlled trial of rasagiline as monotherapy in early Parkinson's disease patients. *Movement Disorders.* 2004; 19(8):916–923. Ref ID: 19854

133 Presthus J, Berstad J, Lien K. Selegiline (1-deprenyl) and low-dose levodopa treatment of Parkinson's disease. A double-blind crossover trial. *Acta Neurologica Scandinavica.* 1987; 76:200–203. Ref ID: 2761

134 Crosby NJ, Deane HO, Clarke CE. Beta-blocker therapy for tremor in Parkinson's disease.(Cochrane Review). *The Cochrane Database of Systematic Reviews.* 2003;(1):CD003361. Ref ID: 80

135 Marsden CD, Parkes JD, Rees JE. Propanolol in Parkinson's disease. *Lancet.* 1974; 2(7877):410. Ref ID: 19533

136 Corbett JL. Beta blockers and the central nervous system. In: Kielkholz P (eds), *An International Symposium,* Bern: Huber, 1976: 200–217. Ref ID: 19534

137 Henderson JM, Yiannikas C, Morris JG et al. Postural tremor of Parkinson's disease. *Clinical Neuropharmacology.* 1994; 17(3):277–285. Ref ID: 755

138 Claveria L, Vakil S, George C et al. Oxprenolol in Parkinsonism. *The Journal of Clinical Pharmacology.* 1975; 15(1):66–68. Ref ID: 19532

139 Crosby N, Deane KHO, Clarke CE. Amantadine in Parkinson's disease (Cochrane Review). *The Cochrane Database of Systematic Reviews.* 2003;(1):CD003468. Ref ID: 51

140 Cox B, Danta G, Schnieden H et al. Interactions of L-dopa and amantadine in patients with Parkinsonism. *Journal of Neurology, Neurosurgery & Psychiatry.* 1973; 36(3):354–361. Ref ID: 19645

141 Savery F. Amantadine and a fixed combination of levodopa and carbidopa in the treatment of Parkinson's disease. *Diseases of the Nervous System.* 1977; 38(8):605–608. Ref ID: 19552

142 Walker JE, Albers JW, Tourtellotte WW et al. A qualitative and quantitative evaluation of amantadine in the treatment of Parkinson's disease. *Journal of Chronic Diseases.* 1972; 25:149–182. Ref ID: 19556

143 Katzenschlager R, Sampaio C, Costa J et al. Anticholinergics for symptomatic management of Parkinson's disease (Cochrane Review). *The Cochrane Database of Systematic Reviews.* 2002;(3): CD003735. Ref ID: 92

144 Cooper JA, Sagar HJ, Doherty SM et al. Different effects of dopaminergic and anticholinergic therapies on cognitive and motor function in Parkinson's disease. *Brain*. 1992; 115(6):1701–1725. Ref ID: 19567

145 Parkes JD, Baxter RC, Marsden CD et al. Comparative trial of benzhexol, amantadine, and levodopa in the treatment of Parkinson's disease. *Journal of Neurology, Neurosurgery & Psychiatry*. 1974; 37(4): 422–426. Ref ID: 19569

146 Hutton JT, Lynne DR, Bianchine JR. Controlled-release carbidopa/levodopa in the treatment of Parkinsonism. *Clinical Neuropharmacology*. 1984; 7(2):135–139. Ref ID: 783

147 Dupont E, Andersen A, Boas J et al. Sustained-release Madopar HBS compared with standard Madopar in the long-term treatment of de novo parkinsonian patients. *Acta Neurologica Scandinavica*. 1996; 93(1):14–20. Ref ID: 778

148 Kinnunen E, Asikaimen I, Jolma T et al. Three-year open comparison of standard and sustained-release levodopa/benserazide preparations in newly diagnosed Parkinsonian patients. *Focus on Parkinson's Disease*. 1997; 9(2):32–36. Ref ID: 304

149 Block G, Liss C, Reines S et al. Comparison of immediate-release and controlled release Carbidopa/Levodopa in Parkinson's disease. A multicenter 5-year study. *European Neurology*. 1997; 37(1):23–27. Ref ID: 257

150 Olanow CW, Hauser RA, Gauger L et al. The effect of deprenyl and levodopa on the progression of Parkinson's disease. *Annals of Neurology*. 1995; 38:771–777. Ref ID: 2746

151 Weiner WJ, Factor SA, Sanchez-Ramos JR et al. Early combination therapy (bromocriptine and levodopa) does not prevent motor fluctuations in Parkinson's disease. *Neurology*. 1993; 43(1):21–27. Ref ID: 2718

152 Rascol O, Brooks DJ, Korczyn AD et al. A five-year study of the incidence of dyskinesia in patients with early Parkinson's disease who were treated with ropinirole or levodopa. *New England Journal of Medicine*. 2000; 342(20):1484–1491. Ref ID: 2540

153 Hely MA, Morris JG, Reid WG et al. The Sydney Multicentre Study of Parkinson's disease: a randomised, prospective five year study comparing low dose bromocriptine with low dose levodopa-carbidopa. *Journal of Neurology, Neurosurgery & Psychiatry*. 1994; 57(8):903–910. Ref ID: 2185

154 Herskovits E, Yorio A, Leston J. Long term bromocriptine treatment in de novo parkinsonian patients. *Medicina*. 1988; 48(4):345–350. Ref ID: 2193

155 Riopelle RJ, Gawel MJ, Libman I et al. A double-blind study of bromocriptine and L-dopa in de novo Parkinson's disease. Short-term results. *European Neurology*. 1988; 28(SUPPL. 1):11–14. Ref ID: 1048

156 Caraceni T, Musicco M. Levodopa or dopamine agonists, or deprenyl as initial treatment for Parkinson's disease. A randomized multicenter study. *Parkinsonism & Related Disorders*. 2001; 7(2):107–114. Ref ID: 324

157 Kulisevsky J, Garcia-Sanchez C, Berthier ML et al. Chronic effects of dopaminergic replacement on cognitive function in Parkinson's disease: a two-year follow-up study of previously untreated patients. *Movement Disorders*. 2000; 15(4):613–626. Ref ID: 2287

158 Holloway RG, Shoulson I, Fahn S et al. Pramipexole vs levodopa as initial treatment for Parkinson disease: a 4-year randomized controlled trial. *Archives of Neurology*. 2004; 61(7):1044–1053. Ref ID: 19842

159 Allain H, Destee A, Petit H et al. Five-year follow-up of early lisuride and levodopa combination therapy versus levodopa monotherapy in de novo Parkinson's disease. *European Neurology*. 2000; 44(1):22–30. Ref ID: 1914

160 Gimenez-Roldan S, Tolosa E, Burguera JA et al. Early combination of bromocriptine and levodopa in Parkinson's disease: a prospective randomized study of two parallel groups over a total follow-up period of 44 months including an initial 8-month double-blind stage. *Clinical Neuropharmacology*. 1997; 20(1):67–76. Ref ID: 2136

161 Alarcon F, Cevallos N, Lees AJ. Does combined levodopa and bromocriptine therapy in Parkinson's disease prevent late motor complications? *European Journal of Neurology*. 1998; 5(3):255–263. Ref ID: 1274

162 Przuntek H, Welzel D, Gerlach M et al. Early institution of bromocriptine in Parkinson's disease inhibits the emergence of levodopa-associated motor side effects. Long-term results of the PRADO study. *Journal of Neural Transmission.* 1996; 103(6):699–715. Ref ID: 2520

163 Ramaker C, Hilten JV. Bromocriptine/levodopa combined versus levodopa alone for early Parkinson's disease. (Cochrane Review). *The Cochrane Database of Systematic Reviews.* 2002;(2):CD003634. Ref ID: 42

164 Hoerger TJ, Bala MV, Rowland C et al. Cost effectiveness of pramipexole in Parkinson's disease in the US. *Pharmacoeconomics.* 1998; 14(5):541–557. Ref ID: 19750

165 Noyes K, Dick AW, Holloway RG. Pramipexole vs levodopa as initial treatment for Parkinson's disease: a randomized clinical-economic trial. *Med Decision Making.* 2004; 24(5):472–485. Ref ID: 19763

166 Iskedjian M, Einarson TR. Cost analysis of ropinirole versus levodopa in the treatment of Parkinson's disease. *Pharmacoeconomics.* 2003; 21(2):115–127. Ref ID: 19745

167 Smala AM, Spottke EA, Machat O et al. Cabergoline versus levodopa monotherapy: a decision analysis. *Movement Disorders.* 2003; 18(8):898–905. Ref ID: 19754

168 Lindgren P, Jonsson B, DuChane J. The cost-effectiveness of early cabergoline treatment compared to levodopa in Sweden. *European Journal of Health Economics.* 2003; 4(1):37–42. Ref ID: 19853

169 Noyes K, Dick AW, Holloway RG. Pramipexole and levodopa in early Parkinson's disease: dynamic changes in cost effectiveness. *Pharmacoeconomics.* 2005; 23(12):1257–1270. Ref ID: 20122

170 Cedarbaum JM, Hoey M, McDowell FH. A double-blind crossover comparison of Sinemet CR4 and standard Sinemet 25/100 in patients with Parkinson's disease and fluctuating motor performance. *Journal of Neurology, Neurosurgery & Psychiatry.* 1989; 52(2):207–212. Ref ID: 261

171 Hutton JT, Morris JL, Bush DF et al. Multicenter controlled study of Sinemet CR vs Sinemet (25/100) in advanced Parkinson's disease. *Neurology.* 1989; 39(11 SUPPL. 2):67–72. Ref ID: 293

172 Hutton JT, Morris JL, Roman GC et al. Treatment of chronic Parkinson's disease with controlled-release carbidopa/levodopa. *Archives of Neurology.* 1988; 45(8):861–864. Ref ID: 295

173 LeWitt PA, Nelson MV, Berchou RC et al. Controlled-release carbidopa/levodopa (Sinemet 50/200 CR4): Clinical and pharmacokinetic studies. *Neurology.* 1989; 39(11 SUPPL. 2):45–53. Ref ID: 310

174 Feldman RG, Mosbach PA, Kelly MR et al. Double-blind comparison of standard Sinemet and Sinemet CR in patients with mild-to-moderate Parkinson's disease. *Neurology.* 1989; 39(11 SUPPL. 2):96–101. Ref ID: 277

175 Lieberman A, Gopinathan G, Miller E et al. Randomized double-blind cross-over study of sinemet-controlled release (CR4 50/200) versus sinemet 25/100 in Parkinson's disease. *European Neurology.* 1990; 30(2):75–78. Ref ID: 157

176 Wolters EC, Horstink MW, Roos RA et al. Clinical efficacy of sinemet CR 50/200 versus sinemet 25/100 in patients with fluctuating Parkinson's disease. An open, and a double-blind, double-dummy, multicenter treatment evaluation. The Dutch Sinemet CR Study Group. *Clinical Neurology & Neurosurgery.* 1992; 94:205–211. Ref ID: 775

177 Wolters EC, Tesselaar HJ. International (NL-UK) double-blind study of Sinemet CR and standard Sinemet (25/100) in 170 patients with fluctuating Parkinson's disease. *Journal of Neurology.* 1996; 243(3):235–240. Ref ID: 19640

178 Sage JI, Mark MH. Comparison of controlled-release Sinemet (CR4) and standard Sinemet (25 mg/100 mg) in advanced Parkinson's disease: A double-blind, crossover study. *Clinical Neuropharmacology.* 1988; 11(2):174–179. Ref ID: 348

179 Juncos JL, Fabbrini G, Mouradian MM et al. Controlled release levodopa-carbidopa (CR-5) in the management of parkinsonian motor fluctuations. *Archives of Neurology.* 1987; 44(10):1010–1012. Ref ID: 109

180 Ahlskog JE, Muenter MD, McManis PG et al. Controlled-release Sinemet (CR-4): a double-blind crossover study in patients with fluctuating Parkinson's disease. *Mayo Clinic Proceedings.* 1988; 63(9):876–886. Ref ID: 248

181   Hammerstad JP, Carter J, Nutt JG. Buspirone in Parkinson's disease. *Clinical Neuropharmacology*. 1986; 9(6):556–560. Ref ID: 401

182   Van Hilten JJ, Ramaker C, van de Beek WJT et al. Bromocriptine for levodopa-induced motor complications in Parkinson's disease (Cochrane Review). *The Cochrane Database of Systematic Reviews*. 1998;(3):CD001203. Ref ID: 47

183   Clarke CE, Deane KH. Cabergoline for levodopa-induced complications in Parkinson's disease (Cochrane Review). *The Cochrane Database of Systematic Reviews*. 2001;(1):CD001518. Ref ID: 52

184   Clarke CE, Speller JM. Lisuride for levodopa-induced complications in Parkinson's disease (Cochrane Review). *The Cochrane Database of Systematic Reviews*. 1999;(1):CD001515. Ref ID: 54

185   Clarke CE, Speller JM. Pergolide for levodopa-induced complications in Parkinson's disease (Cochrane Review). *The Cochrane Database of Systematic Reviews*. 1999;(2):CD000235. Ref ID: 56

186   Clarke CE, Speller JM, Clarke JA. Pramipexole for levodopa-induced complications in Parkinson's disease (Cochrane Review). *The Cochrane Database of Systematic Reviews*. 2000;(2):CD002261. Ref ID: 58

187   Clarke CE, Deane KHO. Ropinirole for levodopa-induced complications in Parkinson's disease (Cochrane Review). *The Cochrane Database of Systematic Reviews*. 2001;(1):CD001516. Ref ID: 60

188   Pogarell O, Gasser T, Van Hilten JJ et al. Pramipexole in patients with Parkinson's disease and marked drug resistant tremor: a randomised, double blind, placebo controlled multicentre study. *Journal of Neurology, Neurosurgery & Psychiatry*. 2002; 72(6):713–720. Ref ID: 2512

189   Wong KS, Lu C-S, Shan D-E et al. Efficacy, safety, and tolerability of pramipexole in untreated and levodopa-treated patients with Parkinson's disease. *Journal of the Neurological Sciences*. 2003; 216(1):81–87. Ref ID: 1823

190   Mizuno Y, Yanagisawa N, Kuno S et al. Randomized, double-blind study of pramipexole with placebo and bromocriptine in advanced Parkinson's disease. *Movement Disorders*. 2003; 18(10):1149–1156. Ref ID: 2405

191   Guttman M, The International Pramipexole-Bromocriptine Study Group. Double-blind comparison of pramipexole and bromocriptine treatment with placebo in advanced Parkinson's disease. *Neurology*. 1997; 49(4):1060–1065. Ref ID: 19602

192   Bateman DN, Coxon A, Legg NJ et al. Treatment of the on-off syndrome in parkinsonism with low-dose bromocriptine in combination with levodopa. *Journal of Neurology, Neurosurgery & Psychiatry*. 1978; 41(12):1109–1113. Ref ID: 19614

193   Gron U. Bromocriptine versus placebo in levodopa treated patients with Parkinson's disease. *Acta Neurologica Scandinavica*. 1977; 56(3):269–273. Ref ID: 19615

194   Maier-Hoehn MM, Elton RL. Low dosages of bromocriptine added to levodopa in Parkinson's disease. *Neurology*. 1985; 35:199–206. Ref ID: 434

195   Jansen EN. Bromocrytine in levodopa response-losing parkinsonism. *European Neurology*. 1978; 17:92–99. Ref ID: 19617

196   Schneider E, Fischer PA. Bromocriptin in der Behandlung der fortgeschrittenen Stadien des Parkinson-syndroms [German]. *Deutsche Medizinische Wochenschrift*. 1982; 107:175–179. Ref ID: 19618

197   Temlett JA, Ming A, Saling M et al. Adjunctive therapy with bromocriptine in Parkinson's disease. *South African Medical Journal*. 1990; 78:680–685. Ref ID: 19620

198   Toyokura Y, Mizuno Y, Kase M et al. Effects of bromocriptine in parkinsonism: a nation-wide collaborative double-blind study. *Acta Neurologica Scandinavica*. 1985; 72:157–170. Ref ID: 19623

199   Miguel F, Obeso JA, Olive Plana JM et al. *Double-blind parallel group study of the efficacy and tolerability of the cabergoline vs placebo in Parkinson's patients with motor fluctuations*. (21336/722i). FCE report, 1993. Ref ID: 19609

200   Steiger MJ, El Debas T, Anderson T et al. Double-blind study of the activity and tolerablility of cabergoline versus placebo in parkinsonains with motor fluctuations. *Journal of Neurology*. 1996; 243:68–72. Ref ID: 19610

201 Hutton JT, Koller WC, Ahlskog JE et al. Multicentre, placebo-controlled trials of cabergoline taken once daily in the treatment of Parkinson's disease. *Neurology.* 1996; 46:1062–1065. Ref ID: 19608

202 Olanow CW, Fahn S, Muenter M et al. A multi-centre double-blind placebo-controlled trial of pergolide as an adjunct to Sinemet in Parkinson's disease. *Movement Disorders.* 1994; 9:40–47. Ref ID: 19607

203 Lieberman A, Ranhosky A, Korts D. Clinical Evaluation of pramipexole in advanced Parkinson's disease: results of a double-blind, placebo-controlled, parallel-group study. *Neurology.* 1997; 49(1):162–168. Ref ID: 19603

204 Pinter MM, Pogarell O, Oertel WH. Efficacy, safety and tolerance of the non-ergoline dopamine agonist pramipexole in the treatment of advanced Parkinson's disease: a double-blind, placebo-controlled, randomised, multi-centre study. *Journal of Neurology, Neurosurgery & Psychiatry.* 1999; 66:436–441. Ref ID: 19604

205 Wermuth L. The Danish Pramipexole Study Group. A double-blind, placebo-controlled, randomised, multi-centre study of pramipexole in advanced Parkinson's disease. *European Journal of Neurology.* 1998; 5:235–242. Ref ID: 19606

206 Rascol O, Lees AJ, Senard JM et al. A placebo-controlled study of ropinirole, a new D2 agonist, in the treatment of motor fluctuations of L-DOPA-treated parkinsonian patients. *Advances in Neurology.* 1996; 69:531–534. Ref ID: 19601

207 Leiberman A, Olanow CW, Sethi K et al. A multicenter trial of ropinirole as adjunct treatment for Parkinson's disease. *Neurology.* 1998; 51:1057–1062. Ref ID: 19612

208 Korcyn AD. *Anti-Parkinson efficacy (L-dopa sparing effect) of ropinirole versus placebo as adjunct therapy in Parkinsonian patients not optimally controlled in L-dopa.* (MY-1002/SKF-101468/2/CPMS-034). SmithKline Beecham Pharmaceuticals, 1990. Unpublished data. Ref ID: 19611

209 Waters CH, Sethi KD, Hauser RA et al. Zydis selegiline reduces off time in Parkinson's disease patients with motor fluctuations: A 3-month, randomized, placebo-controlled study. *Movement Disorders.* 2004; 19(4):426–432. Ref ID: 428

210 Brodersen P, Philbert A, Gulliksen G et al. The effect of l-deprenyl on on-off phenomena in Parkinson's disease. *Acta Neurologica Scandinavica.* 1985; 71:494–497. Ref ID: 2762

211 Presthus J, Hajba A. Deprenyl (selegiline) combined with levodopa and a decarboxylase inhibitor in the treatment of Parkinson's disease. *Acta Neurologica Scandinavica Supplementum.* 1983; 95:127–133. Ref ID: 477

212 Golbe LI, Lieberman AN, Muenter MD et al. Deprenyl in the treatment of symptom fluctuations in advanced Parkinson's disease. *Clinical Neuropharmacology.* 1988; 11(1):45–55. Ref ID: 510

213 Golbe LI, Duvoisin RC. Double-blind trial of R-deprenyl for the "on-off" effect complicating Parkinson's disease. *Journal of Neural Transmission Supplementum.* 1987; 25:123–129. Ref ID: 2760

214 Hubble JP, Koller WC, Waters C. Effects of selegiline dosing on motor fluctuations in Parkinson's disease. *Clinical Neuropharmacology.* 1993; 16:83–87. Ref ID: 2752

215 Sivertsen B, Dupont E, Mikkelsen B et al. Selegiline and levodopa in early or moderately advanced Parkinson's disease: A double-blind controlled short- and long-term study. *Acta Neurologica Scandinavica Supplementum.* 1989; 80(126):147–152. Ref ID: 193

216 Lieberman AN, Gopinathan G, Neophytides A et al. Deprenyl versus placebo in Parkinson disease: a double-blind study. *New York State Journal of Medicine.* 1987; 87:646–649. Ref ID: 88

217 Rascol O, Brooks DJ, Melamed E et al. Rasagiline as an adjunct to levodopa in Parkinson's disease patients with motor fluctuations (LARGO study): a randomised, double-blind, parallel-group trial. *Lancet.* 2005; 365:947–954. Ref ID: 19840

218 Parkinson Study Group. A randomized placebo-controlled trial of rasagiline in levodopa-treated patients with Parkinson disease and motor fluctuations: the PRESTO study. *Archives of Neurology.* 2005; 62(2):241–248. Ref ID: 19833

219 Bonifati V, Meco G. New, selective catechol-O-methyltransferase inhibitors as therapeutic agents in Parkinson's disease. *Pharmacology and Therapeutics.* 1999; 81(1):1–36. Ref ID: 19766

220 Myllyla V, Haapaniemi TH, Kaakkola S et al. New triple combination levodopa/carbidopa/entacapone is a preferred treatment in patients in Parkinson's disease (abstract). *Neurology.* 2003; 60(suppl 1):A289. Ref ID: 20027

221 Deane KHO, Spieker S, Clarke CE. Catechol-O-methyltransferase inhibitors for levodopa-induced complications in Parkinson's disease (Cochrane Review). *The Cochrane Database of Systematic Reviews.* 2004;(4):CD004554. Ref ID: 19624

222 Reichmann H, Boas J, Macmahon D et al. Efficacy of combining levodopa with entacapone on quality of life and activities of daily living in patients experiencing wearing-off type fluctuations. *Acta Neurologica Scandinavica.* 2005; 111(1):21–28. Ref ID: 19864

223 Olanow CW, Kieburtz K, Stern M et al. Double-blind, placebo-controlled study of entacapone in levodopa-treated patients with stable Parkinson disease. *Archives of Neurology.* 2004; 61(10):1563–1568. Ref ID: 104

224 Brooks DJ, Sagar HJ. Entacapone is beneficial in both fluctuating and non-fluctuating patients with Parkinson's disease. A randomized, placebo-controlled, double-blind six month study. *Journal of Neurology, Neurosurgery & Psychiatry.* 2003; 74:1071–1079. Ref ID: 19670

225 Parkinson Study Group. Entacapone improves motor fluctuations in levodopa-treated Parkinson's disease patients. *Annals of Neurology.* 1997; 42(5):747–755. Ref ID: 19637

226 Poewe WH, Deuschl G, Gordin A et al. Efficacy and safety of entacapone in Parkinson's disease patients with suboptimal levodopa response: a 6 month randomised placebo-controlled double-blind study in Germany and Austria (Celomen Study). *Acta Neurologica Scandinavica.* 2004; 105:245–255. Ref ID: 19674

227 Rinne UK, Larsen JP, Siden A et al. Entacapone enhances the response to levodopa in parkinsonian patients with motor fluctuations. Nomecomt Study Group. *Neurology.* 1998; 51(5):1309–1314. Ref ID: 19638

228 Ruottinen HM, Rinne UK. Entacapone prolongs levodopa response in a one month double blind study in parkinsonian patients with levodopa related fluctuations. *Journal of Neurology, Neurosurgery & Psychiatry.* 1996; 60(1):36–40. Ref ID: 19636

229 Fenelon G, Bourdiex I, Pere J, Galiano L, Shadarack J. Entacapone provides additional symptomatic benefits in Parkinson's disease (PD) patients treated with L-DOPA and a dopamine agonist who are experiencing wearing-off motor fluctuations: results of a randomised, double-blind study. AAN conference, 2002. Ref ID: 19671

230 Im JH, Jeon BS, Lee MS et al. A multicentre, double-blind, placebo-controlled study to assess efficacy and safety of entacapone in Korean patients with Parkinson's disease experiencing end-of-dose deterioration. *Movement Disorders.* 2002; 17(5):S40. Ref ID: 19672

231 Myllyla VV, Kultalahti E-R, Haapaniemi H et al. Twelve-month safety of entacapone patients with Parkinson's disease. *European Journal of Neurology.* 2001; 8:53–60. Ref ID: 19673

232 Adler CH, Singer C, O'Brien C et al. Randomized, placebo-controlled study of tolcapone in patients with fluctuating Parkinson disease treated with levodopa-carbidopa. *Archives of Neurology.* 1998; 55(8):1089–1095. Ref ID: 19634

233 Baas H, Beiske A, Ghika J et al. Catechol-O-methyltransferase inhibition with tolcapone reduced the 'wearing-off' phenomenon and levodopa requirements in fluctuating Parkinsonian patients. *Journal of Neurology, Neurosurgery & Psychiatry.* 1997; 63(4):421–428. Ref ID: 19669

234 Dupont E, Burgunder JM, Findley LJ et al. Tolcapone added to levodopa in stable parkinsonian patients: a double-blind placebo-controlled study. *Movement Disorders.* 1997; 12(6):928–934. Ref ID: 19631

235 Kurth MC, Adler CH, Hilaire MS et al. Tolcapone improves motor function and reduces levodopa requirement in patients with Parkinson's disease experiencing motor fluctuations: a multicenter, double-blind, randomized, placebo-controlled trial. Tolcapone Fluctuator Study Group I. *Neurology.* 1997; 48(1):81–87. Ref ID: 19633

236 Myllyla VV, Jackson M, Larsen JP et al. Efficacy and safety of tolcapone in levodopa-treated Parkinson's disease patients with 'wearing-off' phenomenon: A multicentre, double-blind, randomized, placebo-controlled trial. *European Journal of Neurology.* 1997; 4(4):333–341. Ref ID: 19639

237 Rajput AH, Martin W, Saint-Hilaire MH et al. Tolcapone improves motor function in parkinsonian patients with the "wearing-off" phenomenon: a double-blind, placebo-controlled, multicenter trial. *Neurology*. 1997; 49(4):1066–1071. Ref ID: 19632

238 Crosby NJ, Deane HO, Clarke CE. Amantadine for dyskinesia in Parkinson's disease. (Cochrane Review). *The Cochrane Database of Systematic Reviews*. 2003;(2):CD003467. Ref ID: 50

239 Thomas A, Iacono D, Luciano AL et al. Duration of amantadine benefit on dyskinesia of severe Parkinson's disease. *Journal of Neurology, Neurosurgery & Psychiatry*. 2004; 75(1):141–143. Ref ID: 318

240 Luginger E, Wenning GK, Bosch S et al. Beneficial effects of amantadine on L-dopa-induced dyskinesias in Parkinson's disease. *Movement Disorders*. 2000; 15(5):873–878. Ref ID: 152

241 Snow BJ, Macdonald L, Mcauley D et al. The effect of amantadine on levodopa-induced dyskinesias in Parkinson's disease: A double-blind, placebo-controlled study. *Clinical Neuropharmacology*. 2000; 23(2):82–85. Ref ID: 311

242 Verhagen ML, Del Dotto P, van den Munckhof P et al. Amantadine as treatment for dyskinesias and motor fluctuations in Parkinson's disease. *Neurology*. 1998; 50(5):1323–1326. Ref ID: 19594

243 Dewey RB, Hutton JT, LeWitt PA et al. A randomized, double-blind, placebo-controlled trial of subcutaneously injected apomorphine for parkinsonian off-state events. *Archives of Neurology*. 2001; 58(9):1385–1392. Ref ID: 19655

244 Ostergaard L, Werdelin L, Odin P et al. Pen injected apomorphine against off phenomena in late Parkinson's disease: a double blind, placebo controlled study. *Journal of Neurology, Neurosurgery & Psychiatry*. 1995; 58(6):681–687. Ref ID: 19628

245 Van Laar T, Jansen EN, Essink AW et al. A double-blind study of the efficacy of apomorphine and its assessment in 'off'-periods in Parkinson's disease. *Clinical Neurology & Neurosurgery*. 1993; 95(3):231–235. Ref ID: 19992

246 Poewe W, Kleedorfer B, Wagner M et al. Continuous subcutaneous apomorphine infusions for fluctuating Parkinson's disease. Long-term follow-up in 18 patients. *Advances in Neurology*. 1993; 60:656–659. Ref ID: 19651

247 Kanovsky P, Kubova D, Bares M et al. Levodopa-induced dyskinesias and continuous subcutaneous infusions of apomorphine: results of a two-year, prospective follow-up. *Movement Disorders*. 2002; 17(1):188–191. Ref ID: 19656

248 Frankel JP, Lees AJ, Kempster PA et al. Subcutaneous apomorphine in the treatment of Parkinson's disease. *Journal of Neurology, Neurosurgery & Psychiatry*. 1990; 53(2):96–101. Ref ID: 19731

249 Stocchi F, Vacca L, De Pandis MF et al. Subcutaneous continuous apomorphine infusion in fluctuating patients with Parkinson's disease: long-term results. *Neurological Sciences*. 2001; 22(1):93–94. Ref ID: 19733

250 Pietz K, Hagell P, Odin P. Subcutaneous apomorphine in late stage Parkinson's disease: a long term follow up. *Journal of Neurology, Neurosurgery & Psychiatry*. 1998; 65(5):709–716. Ref ID: 19734

251 Hughes AJ, Bishop S, Kleedorfer B et al. Subcutaneous apomorphine in Parkinson's disease: response to chronic administration for up to five years. *Movement Disorders*. 1993; 8(2):165–170. Ref ID: 19735

252 Gancher ST, Nutt JG, Woodward WR. Apomorphine infusional therapy in Parkinson's disease: Clinical utility and lack of tolerance. *Movement Disorders*. 1995; 10(1):37–43. Ref ID: 19737

253 Manson AJ, Turner K, Lees AJ. Apomorphine monotherapy in the treatment of refractory motor complications of Parkinson's disease: long-term follow-up study of 64 patients. *Movement Disorders*. 2002; 17(6):1235–1241. Ref ID: 19730

254 Colzi A, Turner K, Lees AJ. Continuous subcutaneous waking day apomorphine in the long term treatment of levodopa induced interdose dyskinesias in Parkinson's disease. *Journal of Neurology, Neurosurgery & Psychiatry*. 1998; 64(5):573–576. Ref ID: 19736

255 Katzenschlager R, Hughes A, Evans A et al. Continuous subcutaneous apomorphine therapy improves dyskinesias in Parkinson's disease: a prospective study using single-dose challenges. *Movement Disorders*. 2005; 20(2):151–157. Ref ID: 19993

256 Deane KHO, Spieker S, Clarke CE. Catechol-O-methyltransferase inhibitors versus active comparators for levodopa-induced complications in Parkinson's disease (Cochrane Review). *The Cochrane Database of Systematic Reviews.* 2004;(4):CD004553. Ref ID: 19625

257 Koller W, Lees A, Doder M et al. Randomized trial of tolcapone versus pergolide as add-on to levodopa therapy in Parkinson's disease patients with motor fluctuations. *Movement Disorders.* 2001; 16(5):858–866. Ref ID: 307

258 Agid Y, Destee A, Durif F et al. Tolcapone, bromocriptine and Parkinson's disease. *Lancet.* 1997; 350:712–713. Ref ID: 217

259 Lenz FA, Tasker RR, Kwan HC et al. Selection of the optimal lesion site for the relief of parkinsonian tremor on the basis of spectral analysis of neuronal firing patterns. *Applied Neurophysiology.* 1987; 50(1–6):338–43. Ref ID: 19843

260 Cooper IS. Anterior chorodial artery ligation for involuntary movements. *Science.* 1953; 118(3059):193. Ref ID: 19844

261 Laitinen LV, Bergenheim AT, Hariz MI. Leksell's posteroventral pallidotomy in the treatment of Parkinson's disease. *Journal of Neurosurgery.* 1992; 76:53–61. Ref ID: 19845

262 Huntington's Outreach Project for Education at Stanford. *Basal Ganglia.* Available from: www.stanford edu/group/hopes/ [accessed 20 April 2006]. Ref ID: 19939

263 Aziz TZ, Peggs D, Sambrook MA et al. Lesion of the subthalamic nucleus for the alleviation of 1-methyl-4-phenyl-1,2,3,6-tetrahydropyridine (MPTP)-induced parkinsonism in the primate. *Movement Disorders.* 1991; 6(4):288–292. Ref ID: 19846

264 Bergman H, Wichmann T, DeLong MR. Reversal of experimental parkinsonism by lesions of the subthalamic nucleus. *Science.* 1990; 249(4975):1436–1438. Ref ID: 19847

265 Limousin P, Pollak P, Benazzouz A et al. Effect of parkinsonian signs and symptoms of bilateral subthalamic nucleus stimulation. *Lancet.* 1995; 345(8942):91–95. Ref ID: 19848

266 Spottke EA, Volkmann J, Lorenz D et al. Evaluation of healthcare utilization and health status of patients with Parkinson's disease treated with deep brain stimulation of the subthalamic nucleus. *Journal of Neurology.* 2002; 249(6):759–766. Ref ID: 19713

267 Tomaszewski KJ, Holloway RG. Deep brain stimulation in the treatment of Parkinson's disease: A cost-effectiveness analysis. *Neurology.* 2001; 57(4):663–671. Ref ID: 19714

268 McIntosh E, Gray A, Aziz T. Estimating the costs of surgical innovations: The case for subthalamic nucleus stimulation in the treatment of advanced Parkinson's disease. *Movement Disorders.* 2003; 18(9):993–999. Ref ID: 404

269 Charles PD, Padaliya BB, Newman WJ et al. Deep brain stimulation of the subthalamic nucleus reduces antiparkinsonian medication costs. *Parkinsonism & Related Disorders.* 2004; 10(8):475–479. Ref ID: 19708

270 Lagrange E, Krack P, Moro E et al. Bilateral subthalamic nucleus stimulation improves health-related quality of life in PD. *Neurology.* 2002; 59(12):1976–1978. Ref ID: 386

271 Welter ML, Houeto JL, Tezenas du MS et al. Clinical predictive factors of subthalamic stimulation in Parkinson's disease. *Brain.* 2002; 125(3):575–583. Ref ID: 19700

272 Herzog J, Volkmann J, Krack P et al. Two-year follow-up of subthalamic deep brain stimulation in Parkinson's disease. *Movement Disorders.* 2003; 18(11):1332–1337. Ref ID: 19698

273 Funkiewiez A, Ardouin C, Caputo E et al. Long term effects of bilateral subthalamic nucleus stimulation on cognitive function, mood, and behaviour in Parkinson's disease. *Journal of Neurology, Neurosurgery & Psychiatry.* 2004; 75(6):834–839. Ref ID: 19707

274 Tavella A, Bergamasco B, Bosticco E et al. Deep brain stimulation of the subthalamic nucleus in Parkinson's disease: Long-term follow-up. *Neurological Sciences.* 2002; 23(suppl 2):S111–S112. Ref ID: 389

275 Russmann H, Ghika J, Villemure JG et al. Subthalamic nucleus deep brain stimulation in Parkinson disease patients over age 70 years. *Neurology.* 2004; 63(10):1952–1954. Ref ID: 19727

276 Krack P, Batir A, Van Blercom N et al. Five-year follow-up of bilateral stimulation of the subthalamic nucleus in advanced Parkinson's disease. *New England Journal of Medicine.* 2003; 349(20):1925–1934. Ref ID: 19699

277 Limousin P, Speelman JD, Gielen F et al. Multicentre European study of thalamic stimulation in parkinsonian and essential tremor. *Journal of Neurology, Neurosurgery & Psychiatry.* 1999; 66(3): 289–296. Ref ID: 19703

278 Vesper J, Klostermann F, Wille C et al. Long-term suppression of extrapyramidal motor symptoms with deep brain stimulation (DBS). *German Journal of Neurosurgery.* 2004; 65(3):117–122. Ref ID: 400

279 Obeso JA, Guridi J, Rodriguez-Oroz MC et al. Deep-brain stimulation of the subthalamic nucleus or the pars interna of the globus pallidus in Parkinson's disease. *New England Journal of Medicine.* 2001; 345(13):956–963. Ref ID: 417

280 Volkmann J, Allert N, Voges J et al. Safety and efficacy of pallidal or subthalamic nucleus stimulation in advanced PD. *Neurology.* 2001; 56(4):548–551. Ref ID: 19701

281 Ardouin C, Pillon B, Peiffer E et al. Bilateral subthalamic or pallidal stimulation for Parkinson's disease affects neither memory nor executive functions: A consecutive series of 62 patients. *Annals of Neurology.* 1999; 46(2):217–223. Ref ID: 19702

282 Minguez-Castellanos A, Escamilla-Sevilla F, Katati MJ et al. Different patterns of medication change after subthalamic or pallidal stimulation for Parkinson's disease: target related effect or selection bias? *Journal of Neurology, Neurosurgery & Psychiatry.* 2005; 76(1):34–39. Ref ID: 19885

283 Ondo W, Dat VK, Almaguer M et al. Thalamic deep brain stimulation: effects on the nontarget limbs. *Movement Disorders.* 2001; 16(6):1137–1142. Ref ID: 19704

284 Benabid AL, Pollak P, Seigneuret E et al. Chronic VIM thalamic stimulation in Parkinson's disease, essential tremor and extra-pyramidal dyskinesias. *Acta Neurochirurgica Supplement (Wien).* 1993; 58:39–44. Ref ID: 19728

285 Krauss JK, Simpson RK, Jr., Ondo WG et al. Concepts and methods in chronic thalamic stimulation for treatment of tremor: technique and application. *Neurosurgery.* 2001; 48(3):535–541. Ref ID: 19705

286 Karlsen KH, Larsen JP, et al. Influence of clinical and demographic variables on quality of life in patients with Parkinson's disease. *Journal of Neurology, Neurosurgery & Psychiatry.* 1999; 66(4):431–435. Ref ID: 19758

287 Hely MA, Morris JG, Reid J et al. Sydney Multicenter Study of Parkinson's disease: non-L-dopa-responsive problems dominate at 15 years. *Movement Disorders.* 2005; 20(2):190–199. Ref ID: 19892

288 Chaudhuri KR, Schapira A, Martinez-Martin P et al. The holisitic management of Parkinsons' disease using a novel non-motor symptom scale and questionnaire. *Advances in Clinical Neurosciences and Rehabilitation.* 2004; 4:20–24. Ref ID: 19893

289 Goetz CG, Koller WC, Poewe W et al. Treatment of depression in idiopathic Parkinson's disease. *Movement Disorders.* 2002; 17(suppl 4):S112–S119. Ref ID: 19760

290 Schrag A, Jahanshahi M, Quinn N. What contributes to quality of life in patients with Parkinson's disease? *Journal of Neurology, Neurosurgery & Psychiatry.* 2000; 69:308–312. Ref ID: 19887

291 Shabnam G, Chung TH, Deane KHO et al. Therapies for depression in Parkinson's disease (Cochrane Review). *The Cochrane Database of Systematic Reviews.* 2003;(2):CD003465. Ref ID: 78

292 Fregni F, Santos CM, Myczkowski ML et al. Repetitive transcranial magnetic stimulation is as effective as fluoxetine in the treatment of depression in patients with Parkinson's disease. *Journal of Neurology, Neurosurgery & Psychiatry.* 2004; 75(8):1171–1174. Ref ID: 19761

293 Leentjens AF, Vreeling FW, Luijckx GJ et al. SSRIs in the treatment of depression in Parkinson's disease. *International Journal of Geriatric Psychiatry.* 2003; 18(6):552–554. Ref ID: 19762

294 Wermuth L, Sorensen PS, Timm S et al. Depression in idiopathic Parkinson's disease treated with citalopram. A placebo-controlled trial. *Nordic Journal of Psychiatry.* 1998; 52(2):163–169. Ref ID: 19772

295 Andersen J, Aabro E, Gulmann N et al. Anti-depressive treatment in Parkinson's disease. A controlled trial of the effect of nortriptyline in patients with Parkinson's disease treated with L-DOPA. *Acta Neurologica Scandinavica.* 1980; 62(4):210–219. Ref ID: 19771

296 Rabey J, Orlov E, Korczyn A. Comparison of fluvoamine versus amitriptyline for treatment of depression in Parkinson's disease. *Neurology*. (Abstract) 1996; 46:A374. Ref ID: 19788

297 Jiménez-Jiménez FJ, Tejeiro J, Martinez-Junquera G et al. Parkinsonism exacerbated by paroxetine. *Neurology*. 1994; 44(12):2406. Ref ID: 19895

298 Richard IH, Kurlan R, Tanner C et al. Serotonin syndrome and the combined use of deprenyl and an antidepressant in Parkinson's disease. Parkinson Study Group. *Neurology*. 1997; 48(4):1070–1077. Ref ID: 20123

299 Fenelon G, Mahieux F, Huon R et al. Hallucinations in Parkinson's disease: prevalence, phenomenology and risk factors. *Brain*. 2000; 123:733–745. Ref ID: 19888

300 Graham JM, Grunewald RA, Sagar HJ. Hallucinosis in idiopathic Parkinson's disease. *Journal of Neurology, Neurosurgery & Psychiatry*. 1997; 63:434–440. Ref ID: 19889

301 Friedman J, Lannon M, Cornelia C et al. Low-dose clozapine for the treatment of drug-induced psychosis in Parkinson's disease. *New England Journal of Medicine*. 1999; 340(10):757–763. Ref ID: 19775

302 Ondo WG, Levy JK, Vuong KD et al. Olanzapine treatment for dopaminergic-induced hallucinations. *Movement Disorders*. 2002; 17(5):1031–1035. Ref ID: 19778

303 Breier A, Sutton VK, Feldman PD et al. Olanzapine in the treatment of dopamimetic-induced psychosis in patients with Parkinson's disease. *Biological Psychiatry*. 2002; 52(5):438–445. Ref ID: 19776

304 Pollak P, Tison F, Rascol O et al. Clozapine in drug induced psychosis in Parkinson's disease: a randomised, placebo controlled study with open follow up. *Journal of Neurology, Neurosurgery & Psychiatry*. 2004; 75(5):689–695. Ref ID: 19779

305 Ondo W, Tintner R, Dat VK et al. Double-blind, placebo-controlled, unforced titration parallel trial of quetiapine for dopaminergic-induced hallucinations in Parkinson's disease. *Movement Disorders*. 2005; 20(8):958–963. Ref ID: 19933

306 Goetz CG, Blasucci LM, Leurgans S et al. Olanzapine and clozapine: comparative effects on motor function in hallucinating PD patients. *Neurology*. 2000; 55(6):789–794. Ref ID: 264

307 Morgante L, Epifanio A, Spina E et al. Quetiapine and clozapine in parkinsonian patients with dopaminergic psychosis. *Clinical Neuropharmacology*. 2004; 27(4):153–156. Ref ID: 290

308 Ellis T, Cudkowicz ME, Sexton PM et al. Clozapine and risperidone treatment of psychosis in Parkinson's disease. *Journal of Neuropsychiatry & Clinical Neurosciences*. 2000; 12(3):364–369. Ref ID: 19781

309 Bain PG. The management of tremor. *Neurology in Practice*. 2002; 72(5 suppl 1):i3–i9. Ref ID: 2727

310 Message from Professor Gordon Duff, Chairman Committee on Safety of Medicines. *Atypical antipsychotic drugs and stroke*. Available from: www.mhra.gov.uk/home. Date of message: 3 September 2004. Ref ID: 19907

311 Aarsland D, Andersen K, Larsen JP et al. Prevalence and characteristics of dementia in Parkinson's disease: an 8 year prospective study. *Archives of Neurology*. 2003; 60:387–392. Ref ID: 19890

312 Aarsland D, Larsen JP, Karlsen KH et al. Mental symptoms in Parkinson's disease are important contributors to caregiver distress. *International Journal of Geriatric Psychiatry*. 1999; 14:866–874. Ref ID: 19891

313 Emre M, Aarsland D, Albanese A et al. Rivastigmine for dementia associated with Parkinson's disease. *New England Journal of Medicine*. 2004; 351(24):2509–2518. Ref ID: 231

314 Leroi I, Brandt J, Reich S et al. Randomized placebo-controlled trial of donepezil in cognitive impairment in Parkinson's disease. *International Journal of Geriatric Psychiatry*. 2004; 19(1):1–8. Ref ID: 243

315 Pakrasi S, Mukaetova-Ladinska EB, McKeith IG et al. Clinical predictors of response to Acetyl Cholinesterase Inhibitors: experience from routine clinical use in Newcastle. *International Journal of Geriatric Psychiatry*. 2003; 18(10):879–886. Ref ID: 19981

316 Ravina B, Putt M, Siderowf A et al. Donepezil for dementia in Parkinson's disease: a randomised, double blind, placebo controlled, crossover study. *Journal of Neurology, Neurosurgery & Psychiatry*. 2005; 76(7):934–939. Ref ID: 19948

317   Aarsland D, Laake K, Larsen JP et al. Donepezil for cognitive impairment in Parkinson's disease: A randomised controlled study. *Journal of Neurology, Neurosurgery & Psychiatry.* 2002; 72(6):708–712. Ref ID: 19965

318   Giladi N, Shabtai H, Gurevich T et al. Rivastigmine (Exelon) for dementia in patients with Parkinson's disease. *Acta Neurologica Scandinavica.* 2003; 108(5):368–373. Ref ID: 19967

319   Aarsland D, Hutchinson M, Larsen JP. Cognitive, psychiatric and motor response to galantamine in Parkinson's disease with dementia. *International Journal of Geriatric Psychiatry.* 2003; 18(10):937–941. Ref ID: 19958

320   Wild R, Pettit T, Burns A. Cholinesterase inhibitors for dementia with Lewy bodies (Cochrane Review). *The Cochrane Database of Systematic Reviews.* 2003;(3):CD003672. Ref ID: 19787

321   McKeith I, Del Ser T, Spano P et al. Efficacy of rivastigmine in dementia with Lewy bodies: a randomised, double-blind, placebo-controlled international study. *Lancet.* 2000; 356:2031–2036. Ref ID: 208

322   Barone P, Amboni M, Vitale C et al. Treatment of nocturnal disturbances and excessive daytime sleepiness in Parkinson's disease. *Neurology.* 2004; 63(8 (Suppl 3)):S35–S38. Ref ID: 19898

323   Chaudhuri KR, Forbes A, Grosset DG et al. Diagnosing restless legs syndrome (RLS) in primary care. *Current Medical Research Opinion.* 2004; 20(11):1785–1795. Ref ID: 19902

324   Frucht S, Rogers JD, Greene PE et al. Falling asleep at the wheel: motor vehicle mishaps in persons taking pramipexole and ropinirole. *Neurology.* 1999; 52:1908–1910. Ref ID: 19896

325   Adler CH, Caviness JN, Hentz JG et al. Randomized trial of modafinil for treating subjective daytime sleepiness in patients with Parkinson's disease. *Movement Disorders.* 2003; 18(3):287–293. Ref ID: 2780

326   Hogl B, Saletu M, Brandauer E et al. Modafinil for the treatment of daytime sleepiness in Parkinson's disease: a double-blind, randomized, crossover, placebo-controlled polygraphic trial. *Sleep.* 2002; 25(8):905–909. Ref ID: 2781

327   Ondo WG, Fayle R, Atassi F et al. Modafinil for daytime somnolence in Parkinson's disease: double blind, placebo controlled parallel trial. *Journal of Neurology, Neurosurgery & Psychiatry.* 2005; 76(12): 1636–1639. Ref ID: 20116

328   The UK Madopar CR Study Group. A comparison of Madopar CR and standard Madopar in the treatment of nocturnal and early-morning disability in Parkinson's disease. *Clinical Neuropharmacology.* 1989; 12(6):498–505. Ref ID: 19641

329   Ashburn A, Stack E, Pickering RM et al. A community-dwelling sample of people with Parkinson's disease: characteristics of fallers and non-fallers. *Age & Ageing.* 2001; 30:47–52. Ref ID: 19858

330   Schrag A, Ben Shlomo Y, Quinn N. How common are the complications of Parkinson's disease? *Journal of Neurology.* 2002; 294(4):419–423. Ref ID: 19859

331   Wenning GK, Ebersbach G, Verny M et al. Progression of falls in post-mortem-confirmed Parkinsonian disorders. *Movement Disorders.* 2001; 14(6):947–950. Ref ID: 19860

332   Schaafsma JD, Giladi N, Balash Y et al. Gait dynamics in Parkinson's disease:relationship to parkinsonian features, falls and response to levodopa. *Journal of Neurological Sciences.* 2003; 212:47–53. Ref ID: 19861

333   Bloem BR, Grimbergen YA, Cramer M et al. Prospective assessment of falls in Parkinson's disease. *Journal of Neurology.* 2001; 248(11):950–958. Ref ID: 19862

334   Wielinski CL, Erickson-Davis C, Wichmann R et al. Falls and injuries resulting from falls among patients with Parkinson's disease and other Parkinsonian syndromes. Early view published online in advance of print. *Movement Disorders.* 2004;(Dec 3) Ref ID: 19863

335   National Institute for Health and Clinical Excellence. *Falls: The assessment and prevention of falls in older people. Quick reference guide.* (Clinical Guideline 21). London: National Institute for Health and Clinical Excellence, 2004. Ref ID: 20126

336   Abbott R, Cox M, Markus HS et al. Diet, body size and micronutrient status in Parkinson's disease. *European Journal of Clinical Nutrition.* 1992; 46:879–884. Ref ID: 19791

337   Kempster PA, Wahlqvist ML. Dietary factors in the management of Parkinson's disease. *Nutrition Reviews.* 1994; 52:51–58. Ref ID: 19801

338 Gazewood JD, Mehr R. Diagnosis and Management of weight loss in the elderly. *Journal of Family Practice.* 1998; 47(1):19–25. Ref ID: 19934

339 Nilsson H, Ekberg O, Olsson R et al. Quantitative assessment of oral and pharyngeal function in Parkinson's Disease. *Dysphagia.* 1996; 11(2):144–150. Ref ID: 19923

340 Logemann JA, Blonsky ER, Boshe SE. Dysphagia in parkisonism. *Journal of the American Medical Association.* 1975; 231(1):69–70. Ref ID: 19924

341 Hoehn M, Yahr M. Parkinsonism: onset, progression and mortality. *Neurology.* 1967; 17:427–442. Ref ID: 19930

342 Hunter PC, Crameri J, Austin S et al. Response of parkinsonian swallowing dysfunction to dopaminergic stimulation. *Journal of Neurology, Neurosurgery & Psychiatry.* 1997; 63:579–583. Ref ID: 19799

343 Sonies BC. Patterns of care for dysphagic patients with degenerative neurological diseases. *Seminars in Speech and Language Therapy.* 2000; 21:4. Ref ID: 19932

344 Duranceau A. Cricopharyngeal myotomy in the management of neurogenic and muscular dysphagia. *Neuromuscular Disorders.* 1997;(Suppl 1):S85–S89. Ref ID: 19931

345 Pfeiffer RF. Gastrointestinal dysfunction in Parkinson's disease. *Lancet Neurology.* 2003; 2:107–116. Ref ID: 19802

346 Ashraf W, Pfeiffer R, Park F et al. Constipation in Parkinson's disease: objective assessment and response to psyllium. *Movement Disorders.* 1997; 12:946–951. Ref ID: 19793

347 Gruss HJ, Ulm G. Efficacy and tolerability of PEG 3350 plus electrolytes (Movicol) in chronic constipation associated with Parkinson's disease. *European Journal of Geriatrics.* 2004; 6:143–150. Ref ID: 19798

348 Stocchi F, Carbone A, Inghilleri M et al. Urodynamic and neurophysiological evaluation in Parkinson's disease and multiple system atrophy. *Journal of Neurology, Neurosurgery & Psychiatry.* 1997; 62:507–511. Ref ID: 19805

349 Bronner G, Royter V, Korczyn A et al. Sexual dysfunction in Parkinson's disease. *Journal of Sex and Marital Therapy.* 2004; 30:95–105. Ref ID: 19794

350 Singer C, Weiner WJ, Sanchez-Ramos J. Autonomic dysfunction in men with Parkinson's disease. *European Neurology.* 1992; 32:134–140. Ref ID: 19804

351 Allcock LM, Ullyart K, Kenny R et al. Frequency of orthostatic hypotension in a community acquired cohort of patients with Parkinson's disease. *Journal of Neurology, Neurosurgery & Psychiatry.* 2003; 75:1470–1471. Ref ID: 19792

352 Senard JM, Rai S, Lapeyre-Mestre M et al. Prevalence of orthostatic hypotension in Parkinson's disease. *Journal of Neurology, Neurosurgery & Psychiatry.* 1997; 63:584–589. Ref ID: 19803

353 Kaufmann H. Consensus statement on the definition of orthostatic hypotension, pure autonomic failure and multiple system atrophy. *Clinical Autonomic Research.* 1996; 6:125–126. Ref ID: 19800

354 Edwards LL, Pfeiffer R, Quigley E et al. Gastrointestinal symptoms in Parkinson's disease. *Movement Disorders.* 1991; 6:151–156. Ref ID: 19796

355 Boyce HW, Bakheet MR. Sialorrhea: a review of a vexing, often unrecognized sign of oropharyngeal and esophageal disease. *Journal of Clinical Gastroenterology.* 2005; 39(2):89–97. Ref ID: 19936

356 Marks L, Turner K, O'Sullivan J et al. Drooling in Parkinson's disease: A novel speech and language therapy Intervention. *International Journal of Language and Communication Disorders.* 2001; 36(Suppl):282–287. Ref ID: 19922

357 Hyson HC, Johnson AM, Jog MS. Sublingual atropine for sialorrhea secondary to parkinsonism: a pilot study. *Movement Disorders.* 2002; 17(6):1318. Ref ID: 19935

358 Sullivan JD, Bhatia KP, Lees AJ. Botulinum toxin A as a treatment for drooling saliva in PD. *Neurology.* 2000; 55:606–607. Ref ID: 19806

359 Ford B. Pain in Parkinson's disease. *Clinical Neuroscience.* 1998; 5:63–72. Ref ID: 19897

360 Parkinson's Disease Society. *Competencies: an integrated career and competency framework for nurses working in PD management.* London: Parkinson's Disease Society, 2005. Ref ID: 19937

361 Bell L. *Changing roles: the impact of Parkinson's disease nurse specialists.* London: Parkinson's Disease Society, 2004. Ref ID: 787

362 Jarman B, Hurwitz B, Cook A. Effects of community based nurses specialising in Parkinson's disease on health outcome and costs: randomised controlled trial. *British Medical Journal.* 2002; 324(7345): 1072–1075. Ref ID: 223

363 Jahanshahi M, Brown RG, Whitehouse C et al. Contact with a nurse practitioner: A short-term evaluation study in Parkinson's disease and dystonia. *Behavioural Neurology.* 1994; 7(3–4):189–196. Ref ID: 200

364 Reynolds H, Wilson-Barnett J, Richardson G. Evaluation of the role of the Parkinson's disease nurse specialist. *International Journal of Nursing Studies.* 2000; 37(4):337–349. Ref ID: 744

365 Hobson P, Roberts S, Meara J. The economic value of a Parkinson's disease nurse specialist service. *Health and Ageing.* (3); ii–iii. 2003. Ref ID: 19668

366 The Chartered Society of Physiotherapy. *The Curriculum Framework for qualifying programmes in physiotherapy.* London: The Chartered Society of Physiotherapy, The Council for Professions Supplementary to Medicine, 1996. Ref ID: 19660

367 *Physical therapy management of Parkinson's disease (clinics in physical therapy).* New York: Churchill Livingston; 1992. Ref ID: 19678

368 Deane KHO, Jones D, Playford ED et al. Physiotherapy versus placebo or no intervention in Parkinson's disease.(Cochrane Review). *The Cochrane Database of Systematic Reviews.* 2001;(3):CD002817. Ref ID: 90

369 Bergen JL, Toole T, Elliott RG, III et al. Aerobic exercise intervention improves aerobic capacity and movement initiation in Parkinson's disease patients. *NeuroRehabilitation.* 2002; 17(2):161–168. Ref ID: 2778

370 Stallibrass C, Sissons P, Chalmers C. Randomized controlled trial of the Alexander technique for idiopathic Parkinson's disease. *Clinical Rehabilitation.* 2002; 16(7):695–708. Ref ID: 2779

371 Schenkman M, Cutson TM, Kuchibhatla M et al. Exercise to improve spinal flexibility and function for people with Parkinson's disease: a randomized, controlled trial. *Journal of the American Geriatrics Society.* 1998; 46(10):1207–1216. Ref ID: 498

372 Thaut MH, McIntosh GC, Rice RR et al. Rhythmic auditory stimulation in gait training for Parkinson's disease patients. *Movement Disorders.* 1996; 11(2):193–200. Ref ID: 19573

373 Hurwitz A. The benefit of a home exercise regimen for ambulatory Parkinson's disease patients. *Journal of Neuroscience Nursing.* 1989; 21(3):180–184. Ref ID: 415

374 Patti F, Reggio A, Nicoletti F et al. Effects of rehabilitation therapy on Parkinson's disability and functional independence. *Journal of Neurologic Rehabilitation.* 1996; 10(4):223–231. Ref ID: 19572

375 World Federation of Occupational Therapists. *World federation of Occupational therapists definition 2004.* Available from: www wfot com/ [accessed 20 April 2006]. Ref ID: 19869

376 Birleson A. Occupational therapy in Parkinson's disease. *Geriatric Medicine.* 1998; 28(1) Ref ID: 19866

377 Deane HO, Ellis-Hill C, Dekker K et al. A survey of current OT practice for Parkinson's Disease in the UK. *British Journal of Occupational Therapy.* 2003; 66(5):193–200. Ref ID: 19867

378 Aragon A. Physical therapies keep your independence with the help of Occupational therapy. *The Parkinson.* 2004;19–20. Ref ID: 19865

379 Deane KHO, Ellis-Hill C, Playford ED et al. Occupational therapy for Parkinson's disease (Cochrane Review). *The Cochrane Database of Systematic Reviews.* 2001;(2):CD002813. Ref ID: 72

380 Gauthier L, Dalziel S, Gauthier S. The benefits of group occupational therapy for patients with Parkinson's disease. *The American Journal of Occupational Therapy.* 1987; 41(6):360–365. Ref ID: 19739

381 Fiorani CF, Mari F, Bartolini M et al. Occupational therapy increases ADL score and quality of life in Parkinson's disease. *Movement Disorders.* 1997; 121:135. Ref ID: 19738

382 Erb E. Improving speech in Parkinson's disease. *American Journal of Nursing.* 1973; 73:1910–1911. Ref ID: 19877

383   Scott S, Caird FI. Speech Therapy for Parkinson's disease. *Journal of Neurology, Neurosurgery & Psychiatry.* 1983; 47:140–144. Ref ID: 19881

384   Robertson SJ, Thomson F. Speech therapy in Parkinson's disease: a study of the efficacy and long term effects of intensive treatment. *British Journal of Disorders of Communication.* 1984; 19:213–224. Ref ID: 19769

385   Hanson W, Metter E. DAF speech rate modification in Parkinson's disease; a report of two cases. In Berry W (ed), *Clinical disarthria.* Austin, TX: ProEd, 1983:231–254. Ref ID: 19878

386   Rubow R, Swift E. A micro-computer based wearable biofeedback device to improve transfer of treatment in parkinsonian Dysarthria. *Journal of Speech and Hearing Disorders.* 1985; 50:166–178. Ref ID: 19880

387   Deane KHO, Whurr R, Playford ED et al. Speech and language therapy versus placebo or no intervention for dysarthria in Parkinson's disease (Cochrane Review). *The Cochrane Database of Systematic Reviews.* 2001;(2):CD002812. Ref ID: 77

388   Johnson JA, Pring TR. Speech Therapy and Parkinson's disease: A review and further data. *British Journal of Disorders of Communication.* 1990; 25:183–194. Ref ID: 19767

389   Ramig LO, Sapir S, Fox C et al. Changes in vocal loudness following intensive voice treatment (LSVT) in individuals with Parkinson's disease: a comparison with untreated patients and normal age-matched controls. *Movement Disorders.* 2001; 16(1):79–83. Ref ID: 19768

390   Ramig LO, Sapir S, Countryman S et al. Intensive voice treatment (LSVT) for patients with Parkinson's disease: a 2 year follow up. *Journal of Neurology, Neurosurgery & Psychiatry.* 2001; 71(4):493–498. Ref ID: 19770

391   Baumgartner CA, Sapir S, Ramig TO. Voice quality changes following phonatory-respiratory effort treatment (LSVT) versus respiratory effort treatment for individuals with Parkinson disease. *Journal of Voice.* 2001; 15(1):105–114. Ref ID: 20028

392   Sapir S, Ramig LO, Hoyt P et al. Speech loudness and quality 12 months after intensive voice treatment (LSVT) for Parkinson's disease: a comparison with an alternative speech treatment. *Folia Phoniatrica et Logopaedica* 2002; 54(6):296–303. Ref ID: 20029

393   Deane KH, Whurr R, Playford ED et al. Speech and language therapy for dysarthria in Parkinson's disease. *The Cochrane Database of Systematic Reviews.* 2001;(2):CD002814. Ref ID: 20030

394   World Health Organisation. *WHO definition of palliative care.* Available from: www who int/cancer/palliative/definition/en/ [accessed 27 March 2006]. Ref ID: 20127

395   O'Brien T, Welsh J, Dunn FG. ABC of palliative care. Non-malignant conditions. *British Medical Journal.* 1998; 316(7127):286–289. Ref ID: 19938

396   Scott S ,Meadowcroft RS. *Just invisible: a summary.* London: Parkinsons Disease Society, 2005. Ref ID: 19944

397   MacMahon DG, Thomas S. Practical approach to quality of life in Parkinson's disease: the nurse's role. *Journal of Neurology.* 1998; 245(Suppl1):S19–S22. Ref ID: 748

398   MacMahon DG, Thomas S, Campbell S. Validation of pathways paradigm for the management of PD. *Parkinsonism & Related Disorders.* 1999; 5(S53) Ref ID: 19912

399   Parkinson's Disease Society. *Carers' assessment.* (FS46). London: Parkinson's Disease Society, 2003. Ref ID: 19945

400   Buchanan S,Willis E. *Carers' guide.* London: Parkinson's Disease Society, 2004. Ref ID: 19946

401   Goetz CG, Stebbins GT. Risk factors for nursing home placement in advanced Parkinson's disease. *Neurology.* 1993; 43:2227–2229. Ref ID: 19914

402   Goetz CG, Stebbins GT. Mortality and hallucinations in nursing home patients with advanced Parkinson's disease. *Neurology.* 1995; 45:669–671. Ref ID: 19913

403   Mitchell SL, Kiely DK, Kiel DP et al. The epidemiology, clinical characteristics, and natural history of older nursing home residents with a diagnosis of Parkinson's disease. *Journal of the American Geriatrics Society.* 1996; 44(4):394–399. Ref ID: 19915

404   Thomas S, Macmahon D. Parkinson's disease, palliative care and older people: Part 2. *Nursing Older People.* 2004; 16(2):22–26. Ref ID: 19692

405   Thomas S, Macmahon D. Parkinson's disease, palliative care and older people: Part 1. *Nursing Older People.* 2004; 16(1):22–26. Ref ID: 19693

406   Thomas S, Macmahon D. Managing Parkinson's disease in long-term care. *Nursing Older People.* 2002; 14(9):23–30. Ref ID: 20128

407   National Institute for Health and Clinical Excellence. *Pressure relieving devices.* London: National Institute for Health and Clinical Excellence, 2003. Ref ID: 19917

408   National Institute for Health and Clinical Excellence. *Pressure ulcer risk management and prevention (Guideline B).* London: National Institute for Health and Clinical Excellence, 2003. Ref ID: 19916

409   Royal College of Nursing. *Pressure ulcer risk assessment and prevention: implementation guide and audit protocol.* Oxford: Royal College of Nursing, 2003. Ref ID: 19918

410   Howards A, Pemberton C, and Storey L. *The preferred place of care plan (PPC).* Lancashire: Lancashire and South Cumbria Cancer Network, 2004. Ref ID: 19919

411   Macmillan Cancer Relief. *Gold standards framework.* London: Macmillan Cancer Relief, 2005. Ref ID: 19920

412   Liverpool Care Pathway. *Liverpool care pathway for the dying patient.* Liverpool: Liverpool Care Pathway, 2005. Ref ID: 19921

413   Northumbria University, Katholieke Universiteit, Vrije Universiteit. *The rescue project.* Available from: www rescueproject org/overview/welcome/html [accessed on 2 March 2006]. Ref ID: 20121

414   Moher D, Schulz K, Altman D. The CONSORT statement: revised recommendations for improving the quality of reports of parallel-group randomised trials. *Lancet.* 2001; 357:1191–1194. Ref ID: 19448

415   Thomas S, Macmahon D, Maguire J. *Moving and shaping: a guide to commissioning integrated services for people with Parkinson's disease,* 2nd edn. London: Parkinson's Disease Society, 2006. Ref ID: 41

416   Nicholson T, Milne R. *Pallidotomy, thalamotomy and deep brain stimulation for severe Parkinson's disease.* Southampton: Wessex Institute for Health Research and Development, 1999. Ref ID: 43

417   Bhatia K, Brooks DJ, Burn DJ et al. Updated guidelines for the management of Parkinson's disease. *Hospital Medicine (London).* 2001; 62(8):456–470. Ref ID: 9

418   Curtis L, Netten A. *Unit costs of health and social care data 2004.* Personal Social Services Research Unit, University of Kent. Canterbury: 2004. Available from: www.pssru.ac.uk/uc/uc2004.htm